The

Good Mood

Diet

The Good Mood Diet

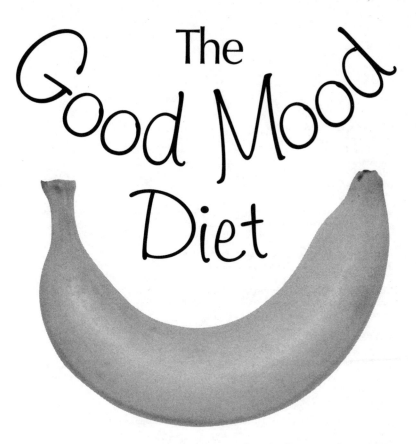

Boost your serotonin levels to lose weight, curb cravings – and feel great!

Judith J. Wurtman, PhD
& Dr Nina Frusztajer Marquis

RODALE

This edition first published in 2007 by
Rodale International Ltd
7–10 Chandos Street
London
W1G 9AD
www.rodalebooks.co.uk

© 2007 by Judith J. Wurtman and Nina Frusztajer Marquis
Published in the US as the Serotonin Power Diet

The moral right of Judith J. Wurtman and Nina Frusztajer Marquis to be identified as the
authors of this work has been asserted in accordance with the Copyright, Design and Patents Act
of 1988.

Printed and bound in the UK by CPI Bath using acid-free paper from sustainable sources.

1 3 5 7 9 8 6 4 2

A CIP record for this book is available from the British Library

ISBN-13: 978-1-4050-9986-8

This paperback edition distributed to the book trade by Pan Macmillan Ltd

Notice

This book is intended as a reference volume only, not as a medical manual. The information given
here is designed to help you make informed decisions about your health. It is not intended as a
substitute for any treatment that you may have been prescribed by your doctor. If you suspect that
you have a medical problem, we urge you to seek competent medical help. Mention of specific
companies, organisations or authorities in this book does not imply endorsement by the publisher,
nor does mention of specific companies, organisations or authorities in the book imply that they
endorse the book.
    Addresses, websites and telephone numbers given in this book were accurate at the time the
book went to press.

To Dick, my husband

– Judith J. Wurtman, PhD

To Camille, Zeno, Hugo and my husband, Andre

– Dr Nina Frusztajer Marquis

'Thou shalt eat and be satisfied.'

– Deuteronomy 11:15

CONTENTS

ACKNOWLEDGEMENTS   ix

INTRODUCTION   xi

Part One: The Brain–Weight Connection

Chapter One: Solving the Carbohydrate Riddle   3

Chapter Two: Appetite, Hunger and Eating Triggers   23

Chapter Three: If You Want to Change Your Weight,
    You Have to Change Your Mind, Too   35

Chapter Four: Before You Begin   49

Part Two: The Programme

Chapter Five: Snack Your Way to Serotonin Power   63

Chapter Six: The Good Mood Diet   74

Chapter Seven: Change Your Body   95

Chapter Eight: Now What Do I Do?   112

Part Three: Planning Your Strategy

Chapter Nine: The 12-Week Guide   133

Chapter Ten: Troubleshooting   155

Chapter Eleven: Maintaining Your Weight Loss   164

Part Four: Cooking the Good Mood Diet

Chapter Twelve: The Kitchen List for a Meal in Minutes   177

Chapter Thirteen: Basic Meals and Quick Kitchen Tricks   181

Chapter Fourteen: Recipes   191

ENDNOTES   259

INDEX   261

ACKNOWLEDGEMENTS

Just as a stool needs three legs to stand on, so too did this book need three writers. The third 'leg' of our writing enterprise was Susan Suffes, who, in a seemingly effortless manner, fused our two writing styles, added her own wisdom and insight to our advice and recommendations, and combed through details and organisational puzzles with endless patience. Her many years as an editor and writer made her an indispensable source of advice and comfort when it looked as if a chapter would drown under the weight of suggested revisions. And her good humour seemed to come from a bottomless supply, which we dipped into without restraint.

The insightful and critical reading of our manuscript by Amy Super, our editor, enabled us to strengthen the book quickly and efficiently. Thank you, Amy, for your constant support and enthusiasm.

We were also amazingly fortunate to work with our agent, Regina Ryan, who, in addition to doing the agent thing, turned out to be a wonderful writer and editor as well. The book benefited substantially from her editorial recommendations and her willingness to try our diet recommendations herself.

Our domestic support was also unfailing: husbands, children, even grandchildren told us constantly how proud they were of our endeavour and gave us the time and support to carry it out.

This book would not be what it is without our many clients, who have given us insight into the complexity of weight gain and the joys and struggles of weight loss. Thank you for your dedication to our programme, your faith in us, and the personal connections we have developed over the years.

Finally, we should thank whoever invented e-mail. We could never have managed our long-distance collaboration so effectively and painlessly without it.

INTRODUCTION

The Good Mood Diet started in a health club in 2001. That's where we met, side by side on elliptical trainers. Between panting and puffing, we learned of our mutual interest and experience in health, weight loss, exercise and diet counselling. Judy was directing a large hospital-based weight-loss clinic, which she had developed, and was contemplating leaving to start a private practice. Nina, a doctor, was deciding how to best tie together her experience as a doctor, nutritionist, lifestyle coach and yoga instructor (and was soon to be a mum).

Our conversations continued beyond the gym and eventually resulted in a private practice called Adara, a Greek name that means beauty. It came from a baby-naming book that Nina was carrying with her at the time.

Adara's mission is to help each client lose weight with the most scientifically advanced programme possible, along with emotional comfort and support. The scientific basis of the Adara programme was founded on years of laboratory research at MIT, followed by reports on hundreds of volunteers who participated in clinical studies. These clinical studies led to the development of a weight-loss plan that included the use of carbohydrate snacks or a carbohydrate drink. After the programme was tested as completely as possible, it became the foundation for a hospital-based weight-loss clinic on the grounds of McLean Hospital in Massachusetts, which opened in 1996. That programme is the one we present to you here, in the Good Mood Diet.

Initially most of our clients had a typical weight-gain history. They put on weight because of lifestyle changes due to marriage, children, jobs, travel and situational stress. These clients responded successfully to the weight-loss programme, which at that time not only included private or group support sessions but also workout time in an on-site gym supervised by the clinic's trainers.

Soon clients began to arrive with an entirely new cause of weight gain. These individuals had been thin all their lives until they were treated with antidepressant and mood-stabilizing drugs. They found themselves gaining weight – in some cases, up to 68 kg (10½ st)!

At the time, there was relatively little known about the potent effect of such drugs on weight gain, and even less was known about how to treat it. The clinic's diet programme, which increased the brain's ability to control appetite, was found to be effective for these clients. They found an almost immediate relief from the incessant carbohydrate cravings induced by the drugs, and they also found they were less tired. Better yet, they began to lose weight and return to their pre-treatment size.

Through our work with these clients, we learned how important it was to combine the effects of the diet programme on the brain with weekly coaching to make people mindful of their personal eating triggers and to teach them strategies to help decrease and eliminate these triggers. In addition, we also stressed the essential role of exercise – not only for their weight loss but also for their general health.

The Good Mood Diet is the same as that followed by our Adara clients. You will be using the same diet plan and experiencing the almost immediate ability to control your appetite and lose your cravings. Those of you who have suffered from emotional overeating will find yourself feeling calm and able to cope with your problems without resorting to eating.

Although we cannot talk with you personally and coach you through the problems that might be causing you to overeat, this book will give you the support you need to stay on the diet – regardless of the stress in your life.

And while we can't exercise with you, we hope that you will take seriously our insistence on the importance of physical activity for weight loss and for your basic health and follow our recommendations.

As you go through the diet programme, you will see positive changes. First you will find yourself feeling full even though you are eating less than before you started the diet. Your mood will improve right away. The people and events that caused you to become upset or angry or impatient or cranky will have much less effect on you.

As your body and mood change, you will also feel energetic and notice an improvement in your stamina and strength.

WHAT TO EXPECT

We know that you are busy. That's why we provide easy-to-follow varied menu plans along with fast and simple recipes for delicious dishes. Carbohydrates are not prohibited or limited. Carbs are essential for weight loss. And of course you will eat protein. Your body needs it. We'll show you how to make the best use of this muscle-building material.

You'll eat real meals and enjoy real snacks. When you go to a restaurant, you won't be stuck; we'll provide plenty of options of what to order. Don't know what to snack on? We're going to give you lots of unexpected and welcome suggestions.

You won't feel deprived. You won't feel your appetite egging you on. You will feel a lot better very quickly and begin to lose fat – not water – fast.

While you must be physically active to lose weight, we're *not* going to demand a long or gruelling daily workout. Instead, we'll give you realistic recommendations that can be integrated into your busy schedule.

The Good Mood Diet is good for you. It is not associated with any adverse health effects; instead, it emphasizes healthy, sustainable lifestyle habits. It will help you to lose 0.5–1 kg (1–2 lb) each week without feeling uncomfortable, agitated or suffering from cravings.

The Good Mood Diet solves the problems of emotional overeating, medication-associated weight gain and post-low-carb diet bingeing. It does so by allowing your brain – and not your willpower – to control your appetite. This means no drugs, no deprivation and no despair.

Instead, you will manage your appetite the way that nature intended you to. The strategy for weight loss, followed by a lifetime of weight control, is finally in your hands.

Our best wishes for an easy journey to your weight goal. Our thoughts are with you.

Judith J. Wurtman, PhD

Dr Nina Frusztajer Marquis

PART ONE

THE BRAIN–WEIGHT CONNECTION

Solving the Carbohydrate Riddle

Eating carbs and losing weight seem like opposites that never attract. How can you eat the carbohydrates you love when you hate the weight you gain when you eat carbohydrates?

This love-hate relationship often dictates how you try to lose weight. You avoid carbohydrates by going on a high-protein diet. When you go off the diet, carbohydrates are the first foods you reach for and you overeat. Or, when you are stressed, all of your good intentions to watch your carbohydrate intake are tossed aside. It's as though an uncontrollable force pulls you towards anything that is sweet or starchy – or both. As the stress mounts and the weight piles on, you feel powerless to stop eating the carbohydrates. What are you supposed to do?

Maybe you never had a weight problem until, like millions of others, you began to take antidepressants. For a reason you can't fathom, you never feel full, no matter how much you eat. Suddenly carbohydrates are the only food you really want. And as you give in to this new craving, your weight goes up. What are you supposed to do?

At last there is an answer, based on decades of research and clinical experience. You must eat carbohydrates to lose weight and you must eat carbohydrates to maintain the loss.

THE CARBOHYDRATE–SEROTONIN CONNECTION

As hard as it may be to believe, carbohydrates are as essential for weight loss as petrol is to a car. They not only drive the system that controls appetite, they also control emotional eating and mood.

3

At this point many of you who have been told that the road to weight ruin is paved with carbohydrates (especially the yummy ones) are likely reading this in disbelief. How can it be? Don't carbs bulk up fat cells? Shouldn't they be avoided, or at least limited to brown rice, a few leafy vegetables and occasionally some fruit? How can it be possible to eat pasta, potatoes, rice and even bread if you want to lose weight? And how can you stop overeating carbohydrates once you start?

It is not only possible to eat carbohydrates and lose weight, it is essential to do so. The reason lies within your brain.

Eating carbohydrates triggers a process involving the hormone insulin, an amino acid called tryptophan, and a barrier between the blood and the brain. The net result of this process is the production of a brain chemical called serotonin.

Serotonin is the switch that turns off your appetite. It is the 'I have had enough to eat' switch. Serotonin is also the control that restores your good mood after minor and major stresses erode it. When produced consistently and regularly, serotonin prevents the tendency to eat impulsively when stresses occur.

Nature seems to have tagged serotonin as the only food-dependent brain chemical. At the same time, nature did you an enormous favour. By being able to manufacture serotonin by eating sweet or starchy carbohydrates, you can tap into a built-in appetite suppressant and mood regulator.

That's why the Good Mood Diet is based on maximizing serotonin production. Our carbohydrate-friendly, serotonin-producing diet will satisfy your appetite even though you will be eating fewer calories. If antidepressants are making you overeat, our diet will give you control over your appetite. It will take away the mental fatigue that keeps you from exercising. And the Good Mood Diet will also buffer you when you respond to stresses that otherwise would have you setting a world record for hand-to-mouth eating.

UNDERSTANDING CARBOHYDRATES

Carbohydrates come in two basic forms: simple and complex. The simple ones, also called sugars (as in table sugar, or sucrose, and milk sugar, or lactose), are made up of one or two molecules. They are digested very quickly into the simplest carbohydrate of all, glucose.

Glucose, which circulates in the blood, is the sugar used by muscles for energy. When you exercise, your muscles use a stored form of carbohydrate called glycogen. Marathon runners 'carbo-load' before a race to increase the amount of glycogen in their muscles.

Complex carbohydrates are made up of the same molecules, but in long chains with branches. You know these carbohydrates as starches and eat them as potatoes, pasta, bread, cereal, rice, oats, barley, millet, rye and other grains. Beans and lentils, although higher in protein than some other carbohydrates, are also included in this family of starches. Complex carbohydrates are also digested into the simplest carbohydrate, glucose, but it takes longer for them to reach this state because of their complexity.

Thus, all carbohydrates end up as glucose as soon as they leave the intestines and enter the bloodstream. Fruits, which contain fructose, are the exception. Fructose must go through an additional biochemical process in order to be converted into glucose.

SCIENCE EXPLAINS THE BRAIN–SEROTONIN CONNECTION

At the Massachusetts Institute of Technology (MIT) in the 1970s, Dr Richard Wurtman (Judy's husband) and one of his students made groundbreaking discoveries about the connection between the brain, serotonin and carbohydrates. They discovered that after animals ate carbohydrates, their brains contained more serotonin.[1-4]

The connection between carbohydrates and serotonin was puzzling and quite unexpected. It was already known that serotonin is made when the amino acid tryptophan enters the brain. It was also known that tryptophan is one of many amino acids that make up protein. For instance, tryptophan is found in protein foods such as steak, fish, chicken and eggs. Tryptophan is not found in carbohydrate foods such as potatoes, bread and pasta. So it seemed logical that eating protein, not a carbohydrate, would prompt serotonin production.

But that's not what happened. When laboratory rats were fed a protein meal (such as the protein in milk), their brains made no new serotonin. And when protein was added to a meal containing carbohydrate, no serotonin was made either, even though the rats were eating carbohydrate. It seemed as if eating protein prevented serotonin from being made.

After the scientific equivalent of 'Huh?' was exclaimed, the research team examined how tryptophan gets into the brain from the bloodstream. They knew that there is a barrier around the brain that controls what actually enters the brain from the bloodstream. Some of the substances the brain needs enter through certain 'doorways'. It was known that tryptophan enters the brain through a particular doorway along with a group of amino acids called neutral amino acids. These amino acids compete with each other to get into the brain through this door the way shoppers compete with each other to be the first ones in the shops for the January sales. The bloodstream fills up with amino acids after protein is eaten and digested. So it seems logical that this would be when a lot of tryptophan gets into the brain. But just the opposite happens. Very little tryptophan gets into the brain because there is less tryptophan in protein than there are other amino acids. So when the amino acids cluster around the doorway to the brain, the larger number of neutral amino acids squeeze tryptophan out and send it to the back of the crowd. Although some tryptophan may get into the brain, it is not enough to make new serotonin.

This still left the question, How does tryptophan get into the brain so easily after carbohydrate is eaten? It is as if the manager of the shop plucks tryptophan from the back of the crowd and sends it through the doorway first.

When any carbohydrate is eaten, with the exception of fruit, the hormone insulin is released from the pancreas. (Only trivial amounts of insulin are released in response to dietary fructose.) As digested glucose enters the bloodstream, insulin sends it into the organs of the body, where it is used as energy. Within several minutes the level of glucose in the blood returns to pre-meal levels.

As insulin pushes the glucose into the organs, it also sends amino acids out of the blood into the organs. Tryptophan is also sent away – but not as fast as the other amino acids. Think of that crowd in front of the shop. The people pushing to get in melt away, leaving only one person to walk easily through the doorway. Tryptophan no longer has any difficulty getting into the brain. Once in the brain, it is quickly converted into serotonin.

Dr Richard Wurtman, Judy and their colleagues concluded after further research that eating carbohydrate is the only way tryptophan can get into the brain to make serotonin.

Why is this important for you to know? Because, as Judy's later research found, as serotonin is made it begins to turn off your appetite and make you content with eating less. It turns on your good mood and makes you resistant to stress-triggered overeating. And serotonin can make you feel more energetic.

THE SEROTONIN–APPETITE CONNECTION

It wasn't always obvious that serotonin is involved in regulating eating. People used to believe that when the stomach filled up, eating would stop. (Of course anyone who has happily consumed a portion of dessert despite feeling stuffed from the main course would dispute this assumption.)

After the initial serotonin studies were completed, Judy and her colleagues at MIT conducted further research to determine if cravings for sweet and starchy foods were related to serotonin and carbohydrates.

The work was not done in isolation; much research done elsewhere in the United States and in Europe showed that the brain contained the master switch to turn off eating.

Judy's first set of studies on laboratory animals showed that when brain serotonin was made more active, the animals stopped eating.[5–7] After animals were treated with drugs that increased serotonin's activity, their food intake was compared to that of animals treated with a placebo.

The treated animals stopped eating much sooner than the animals who were not given these drugs. This was not an isolated result – these studies were done many times to make sure that the results were valid. It was very exciting to find that the brain, and not the full stomach, was able to turn off eating.

Then Judy's team wondered what would happen if animals did not have enough serotonin in their brains. Normally, laboratory animals eat a great deal of carbohydrate, so presumably their brains were able to make new serotonin at any time. Would the animals eat differently if their daily carbohydrate were taken away from them? Would the absence of carbohydrate and the absence of serotonin have any effect on how much they ate? Might they exhibit the animal version of a binge?

To find out, rats were given the same number of calories they usually received, but the food contained only protein and fat. They were not allowed to eat any carbohydrate. The rats stayed on this rodent version of the Atkins Diet for 3 weeks. Other rats were given normal rat food, which contained carbohydrate as well as protein and fat, for the same period of time. After the 3 weeks were over, both groups were given three dishes of food. One dish contained protein, the second held fat and the third contained a mixture of starch and sugar.

The rats that had been allowed to eat carbohydrates in the previous 3 weeks continued to do so, taking a small amount of food from all three dishes.

Things were different for the carbohydrate-deprived rats. They binged on the carbohydrates, ignoring the protein and fat. Rats normally do not binge. Rats always control what they eat. Something had happened.

The research team found that there was very little tryptophan or serotonin in the rats' brains. The few weeks of a no-carbohydrate diet had prevented serotonin from being made. And as a result, not only were the animals eating more than they usually ate, they were actually seeking out carbohydrate. Was the brain telling them what to eat to restore depleted serotonin levels?

If so, the brain succeeded in this case. By the next day the formerly carbohydrate-starved rats were eating as they had before the experiment. It seemed that their serotonin levels were back to normal.

But could the same also be true of people? Would their serotonin levels and their eating also be affected by the lack of carbohydrates? To find out, human volunteers at MIT were recruited to go on a carbohydrate-free diet. Their blood was tested for amino acid levels that would tell whether serotonin was or wasn't being made in their brains.

The findings were not surprising. The blood tests on the volunteers confirmed that very little tryptophan could get into the brain to make new serotonin. And the lack of serotonin had an impact on how the volunteers felt. They craved carbohydrates constantly and complained about not feeling full, even though they were getting more than enough food.

But scientists have to be sceptical. Maybe the volunteers just missed the tastes and textures of carbohydrates, which would explain why they grumbled about not feeling satisfied. It might not have been due to the lack of serotonin at all.

The only way to tell whether their feelings of deprivation were caused by their brains or their taste buds was to change serotonin activity in their brains without telling them.

It was decided to see if the volunteers still had their cravings when serotonin activity was increased in the brain with a research drug. The volunteers were given either a test medication or a placebo without their knowing which treatment they were taking. If their cravings for carbohydrate decreased after being treated with the test drug and they felt as satisfied as they would have if they had eaten, the researchers could be reasonably sure that these feelings were due to changes in serotonin and not taste buds.

Several studies showed that volunteers treated with the placebo did not experience any decrease in their appetite or carbohydrate cravings. On the other hand, the volunteers who were treated with the test medication experienced decreased carbohydrate cravings. One volunteer said, 'I used to polish off the leftovers before they were carried to the kitchen. But for a couple of weeks I couldn't even finish what was on my plate. I learned later that those were the weeks when I was taking the drug.'

These experiments, and others like them, suggested that serotonin is the key to controlling appetite so that people can stick to the portion sizes of a diet without difficulty. Serotonin is also the key to minimizing cravings for sweet and starchy snack foods, the downfall of many a dieter.

And nature revealed the perfect diet tool to manipulate serotonin: carbohydrates. To lose weight, no drugs, supplements or strange food combinations – or side effects – are necessary. Carbohydrate snacks, however, are welcome.

SNACKS: YOUR UNEXPECTED ALLY

From the studies' conclusions, we guessed that carbohydrate snacks would help control appetite, reduce cravings, and prevent overeating when emotionally upset. Before making the snacks an essential part of the Good Mood Diet, we tested our theory.

Studies were done with obese volunteers who wanted to lose weight. All of the volunteers were told they would be given one of two drinks that contained the same number of calories. One was composed solely of carbohydrate and the other contained carbohydrate and protein. They were told that one drink would increase serotonin and might cut back their appetite and food intake while the other was unlikely to have any impact.

To disguise the drinks so that neither the volunteers nor the people giving them the drinks knew what they contained, the research dietician concocted beverages that looked and tasted identical.

The volunteers consumed one drink an hour before lunch and a second drink an hour before dinner. At the end of the study, the amount of weight loss was measured. It turned out that the volunteers who were given the carbohydrate drink lost more weight and found it easier to stay on the diet than the volunteers whose drink contained a mixture of protein and carbohydrate.

Another study used the same methodology with female volunteers who suffered from mood changes when they had PMS. Judy had earlier discovered that PMS mood changes were due to changes in the action of serotonin, so it wasn't surprising when the carbohydrate beverage improved the women's moods. In addition, the women who drank the carbohydrate beverage experienced reduced carbohydrate cravings.

This drink was eventually manufactured for use in the hospital weight-loss clinic that Judy began in 1996. The drink was called Serotrim. (Although at the time of going to press, the drink is only available in the US, there are plans to make it more widely available.)

Although Serotrim was used in these studies, a large number of snack foods were identified that were similar to the drink in carbohydrate content. The clients at the clinic, and later at Adara, were given a choice of using the beverage or something from a long list of snacks. Many people decided to snack, whereas others used the drink at the beginning of the diet because it was easier to fit into their schedule or because the pre-measured drink took away their fear that they would overeat with the snacks. No one ever overindulged in the drink.

Snacks containing the same amount of carbohydrate as the drink will work just as well to decrease appetite and control how much is being eaten. That exact amount determined by Judy's research studies is provided for you in the Good Mood Diet.

Miriam, a single mum who worked from home and struggled with her weight for years, knew all about carbohydrate overloading. She kept only healthy snacks in the house, but she also kept, in her words, a healthy appetite for them.

'If I start to snack on wholegrain crackers, I can finish the box while working at the computer,' she related. 'I don't even notice how much I am eating until the box is empty. So most of the time, I refuse to allow myself any carbohydrates because of my lack of control. Once I give in and start to snack, I've bought a one-way ticket to a binge state.'

When Miriam started on the diet plan, she preferred using Serotrim to carbohydrate snacks because she knew the drink would not be a bingeing trigger. After about a week on the drink, she became very sensitive to the feeling of satisfaction and calmness that followed its consumption. Then she experimented with daily carbohydrate snacks that did not tempt her. Bread sticks, oatmeal and shredded wheat squares were her choices.

By the end of the second week Miriam no longer felt a compulsion to eat carbohydrates. Nor did eating a small amount create any problems. Her previous tendency to binge, which always followed a period of carbohydrate deprivation, had vanished. In its place was the ability to enjoy a carbohydrate snack and then stop and wait the 20 minutes or so for the effects to be felt.

'I feel like a different person,' she said. 'And the fact that I can control the carbs I eat is nothing less than astounding.'

ACTIVATE YOUR APPETITE-CONTROL SWITCH

This is the way it works: eat carbohydrates before a meal, and serotonin is boosted. Serotonin works naturally to turn off appetite. The effect? Eat less and be more satisfied.

You've already done it on many occasions. Haven't you gone to a restaurant and eaten bread rolls or bread sticks while waiting for your meal to arrive? How often did you say when the food was served, 'I'm not really hungry anymore'? Of course you still ate – but the carbohydrates that you nibbled on earlier took the edge off of your appetite. The calories were not sufficient to take away your appetite. Rather, it was the serotonin produced by eating the carbohydrates that began to make you feel full.

The Good Mood Diet taps into the power of carbohydrates to

activate your built-in appetite switch. You will be satisfied with the portions on the diet and you won't feel like eating more. And the serotonin appetite-control switch will continue working after the completion of your diet, as long as you keep eating carbohydrates. Your appetite will be controlled and so will your weight.

Perhaps you are sceptical. Could so simple a technique work? Perhaps you've never been able to control your carbohydrate intake. Martha, a client and veteran of every popular diet trend of the last 30 years, didn't believe it, either.

A 55-year-old financial analyst, Martha said, 'I cannot stay on a diet, and I have tried them all. My problem is that after a few weeks, no matter how much I am eating, I am never satisfied. I am not hungry, but I want to eat more. Eventually, I start eating larger and larger portion sizes. Then the snacking starts, on carbohydrates of course. Soon, it's bye-bye, diet.'

None of the programmes Martha had tried allowed her to eat more than a small portion of carbohydrates, and then only as a side dish. Snacks, when they were allowed, were limited to fruit and fat-free yogurt.

We told Martha about serotonin switching off her appetite so her brain would give her a feeling of fullness. Dubious and even a little fearful when informed that she would be eating carbohydrate snacks before lunch, late in the afternoon, and again, for the first few weeks, in the evening, she replied, 'I'll never be able to lose weight on your diet. Still, I love the choices, especially all the carbohydrates at dinner. Even if I don't lose weight, at least I'll be a happy eater.'

Two weeks later an ecstatic Martha was 2.2 kg (5 lb) lighter. 'This is the easiest diet I have ever tried,' she admitted. 'I just don't feel like eating. I actually force myself to finish my dinner; I think you are giving me too much food. And the feelings of satisfaction and being content are, so to speak, the icing on the cake.'

But Martha, being an analyst, still had some questions.

'I know I shouldn't complain, but when I went on the no-carb diet, I dropped 2.7 kg [6 lb] the first week. Why am I losing more slowly?'

The explanation was that low- or no-carbohydrate diets allow the body to lose water very quickly, as the carbohydrate stored in muscle, along with water, is used up. In stark contrast, the Good Mood Diet, which contains normal amounts of carbohydrates, doesn't work that way. The weight loss seen on the scales is from shrinking fat cells, not water loss.

Finally, Martha wanted to know, 'Will I have to follow the diet for the rest of my life?' The answer was no.

But there was a caveat. If she began avoiding carbohydrates, her serotonin levels would start to drop, leaving her with a dissatisfied appetite and a less-than-good mood. To keep the serotonin system running optimally, she has to eat carbohydrates every day, not eat more on one day and none the next. It is no different from drinking water. A glass drunk today cannot relieve tomorrow's thirst.

CARBS EVERY DAY KEEP THE CRAVINGS AWAY

When your body needs water, the urge to drink overwhelms all other needs and behaviours. Once that need is satisfied, the urge disappears and you feel so much better. You would never avoid drinking water because a diet plan suggested you do so to weigh less.

Avoiding carbohydrates to lose weight makes about as much sense. Your brain needs you to eat carbohydrate to make serotonin. It signals you to do so by making you feel a desire to eat sweet or starchy foods. Just as eating crackers cannot quench thirst, neither can protein or fatty foods meet the brain's need for you to eat carbohydrates. And just as your body turns off thirst when you drink enough water, when you ingest enough carbohydrates, your carbohydrate cravings disappear. And just as important, your appetite-control system functions optimally. But if you neglect to eat enough carbohydrate or drink enough water, the intense urge to eat or drink will stay with you until you do so.

Wait a minute, you may be thinking. Your brother or boss or friend claimed that his or her hunger was controlled completely by protein and fat. You know people who avoid carbohydrates and who cannot understand why others complain about the lack of carbohydrates. When stressed, these dieters eat fatty foods instead. (We once had a client who ate mayonnaise when she was anxious. She said the fat made her so tired she did not have to think about her problems.)

USE THE REAL THING

Both sugar and starch or one or the other allow the brain to make serotonin. However, sugar substitutes, even though they taste sweet, will not make serotonin. You cannot fool Mother Nature.

So how do we explain successful dieters who shun carbohydrates and lose weight without the help of serotonin?

Yes, it is possible to lose weight by eating only protein and fat. And it is feasible to deal with stress by eating lots of high-fat foods like chocolate, cheese and ice cream. The stomach, as it is filled, helps to control food intake by being stretched. Additionally, if the food leaves the stomach very slowly, the stomach feels full for a long time. When this happens, the person feels stuffed.

High-fat and high-protein foods empty slowly from the stomach and small intestine. This is why foods like bacon, beef, butter, eggs, mayonnaise and whipped cream produce a feeling of fullness that lasts a long time.

Over the first several weeks of a low- or no-carb diet, the novelty of eating eggs topped with cheese and bacon or a large steak every day wears off and the dieter automatically tends to eat less and, therefore, loses weight.

But what happens if, in the interest of good health and nutrition, the dieter begins to cut back on the fat and protein and starts adding vegetables, fruit, low-fat dairy products and high-fibre carbohydrates to meals? Disaster! During the diet, the serotonin hunger-control system was rendered ineffective and now the stomach empties too quickly to keep a person satisfied with small portion sizes. At this point, many people feel unable to stay on a low-fat diet and quickly revert back to the high-fat, high-protein regime.

Moreover, the strong signal sent by the brain to eat more and more carbohydrates adds to the dieter's distress. The brain is like a lost soul in the Sahara finding an oasis after days of sand and thirst. Just as the traveller will drink and drink, the carbohydrate-deprived dieter will eat and eat carbohydrates. And therein lies the reason so many dieters distrust carbohydrates.

'I took myself off of the high-protein, high-fat diet and allowed myself a half a bagel. Big mistake. I ate two whole ones right afterward,' a lapsed high-protein, high-fat dieter who is now a client confessed. 'Now I feel like a carb addict and I'm afraid to go near them again.'

Is carbohydrate bingeing inevitable? No, it's not. The Good Mood Diet approach is basic. You must eat carbohydrates, in the right amounts and at the right times, every day. When you do so, your brain won't force you to binge.

THE PROTEIN PREDICAMENT

While protein is a necessary nutrient and a significant component of the Good Mood Diet, relying on protein and drastically limiting carbohydrates in the interest of cutting calories may leave your brain seeking, but not finding, enough serotonin. The scientific facts are clear. No serotonin is produced if you eat:

- Protein alone
- Fat and protein together
- A serving of protein along with a serving of carbohydrate

But nothing is as simple as it seems, since eating small amounts of protein along with much larger amounts of carbohydrate will still allow tryptophan to enter the brain easily. (This information came from long

MEN, WOMEN, AND THE NEED FOR SEROTONIN

A woman once defined hell as wearing tights every day, having a husband who is always flicking the TV remote, and being on a no-carbohydrate diet.

As one of our female clients related, 'I was on low-carb diet for all of 3 days when I felt I was spiralling into total meltdown. As my mood plummeted, my carb cravings reached an all-time high, and I obsessed about anything made with flour. My mood was so awful that my colleagues suggested that I relocate my desk – permanently. By day 4, the diet plan was in the bin and I was digging into a pot of pasta.'

Women feel the absence of carbohydrate more acutely than men do because women's brains synthesize 50 per cent less serotonin.[8]

This difference may help to explain why women are more prone to mood disorders such as depression, which involve a lack of serotonin activity. It is also possible that these lower serotonin levels render a woman more sensitive to the effect of minor stresses on her mood and the accompanying urge to eat carbohydrates to increase serotonin.

Though men can tolerate a high-protein, high-fat diet for longer periods of time, they will eventually feel the effects of serotonin depletion, too.

and laborious MIT research on laboratory animals that ate the equivalent of different amounts of mashed potatoes with different amounts of turkey.) We used this knowledge to build the serotonin-optimizing meal plans you'll find in Chapter 6.

SEROTONIN: THE BRAIN'S MOOD ELEVATOR

When the research teams at MIT started to look at the link between emotions, eating carbohydrate and serotonin, it was assumed that carbohydrate eaters had improved moods because of the taste, texture or mouth feel of the food. But that theory didn't explain why, after the food has been swallowed and the taste goes away, the better mood is still there (although it may be seasoned with guilt).

So why the improvement in mood? The brain manufactured more serotonin, which, in its other role as a natural antidepressant, relieved some of the unpleasant sensations associated with stress.

Sandra, a client, was a typical stressed overeater. She ate at night after leaving her 16-hour-a-day, 6-day-a-week crisis-filled job. Although she managed to keep her eating under control during the day, mainly because she was never alone, her evenings were a snack-food free-for-all.

'I am the poster child of carb craving,' she confessed. 'I will eat anything as long as it is a carbohydrate: jelly beans, crisps, crackers, gumdrops, even sugar out of the container. No matter how much I try I can't stop myself. The only time I feel relaxed and can turn off my constant obsessing about work is after I've gotten my fill of carbs. After a particularly stressful day, I can't wait to get home and start eating. Only afterward can I calm down.'

Sandra, like many of our clients, used carbohydrates as edible tranquilizers. She is not alone. Emotional distress – or even a surge of positive emotion – is a potent force that pushes people to eat. That's because food alters mood. While food is not a drug and cannot deliver either the effectiveness or staying power of a tranquilizer or antidepressant, it does soothe, take the edge off anxiety, increase focus and coping skills and alleviate fatigue associated with stress. When the brain increases the serotonin level after carbohydrates have been eaten, there is a feeling of emotional relief.

Unfortunately, when food is eaten as a tranquilizer it does not come with a warning label. High-fat foods like pastries and ice cream and chocolate do not provide this caution: 'Do not eat when under extreme stress. Overdosing on calories is a common side effect.'

Consequently, like Sandra, many of our clients in our weight-loss practice suffer the side effects of either eating too much food or using the wrong kinds of food to give them emotional comfort.

Jane gained 11.3 kg (1¾ st) because she could not break up with her abusive boyfriend. After every horrible encounter she downed a large tub of premium ice cream with a large chocolate bar chaser. She finally broke up with him for good before all of her clothes stopped fitting.

Martin was already suffering the health consequences of the 40-odd extra kilograms (6 st) he could not lose. Facing a potential company bankruptcy, the 60-something CEO stuffed himself with snacks from the company kitchen from 8 a.m. Monday to 7 p.m. Friday to quell his business anxieties.

As a single mum, Phyllis's diets ended every time she had to deal with her adopted son's multiple learning disorders and emotional problems. Only by eating a packet of biscuits every night could she find the necessary patience.

Larry was a soloist in a church choir. He attributed his extra weight to the half-dozen or more doughnuts and pastries he downed after the service. It was the only way he could lower his adrenalin after the performance to help him with his schoolwork.

All of these people were responding appropriately to their brain's need to restore emotional balance by eating carbohydrates. But their weight gain reflected their inability to choose the right carbohydrates, much less the correct amounts.

If you make a beeline for carbohydrates whenever your emotions are shaken, your brain is sending you to these foods. Your stress is triggering a need for more serotonin, and if you listen to your brain and eat the carbohydrates, the increase in serotonin will calm you. Instinctively, you are doing the right thing.

But beware. Many people under stress gravitate toward carbohydrates that also contain a lot of fat, like gourmet ice cream, crisps, doughnuts, biscuits and chocolate. The high-fat ingredients certainly improve the taste of the food. But the fat may do more than soothe you;

it can turn you into an emotional zombie. Moreover, the calorie content of these fatty foods is so high that they're all but incompatible with weight-loss goals.

There is yet another reason to avoid these foods. They take too long to work. If the carbohydrate snack is high in fat, it takes much longer to be digested and that much longer for serotonin to be made. Why wait so long? If you are in emotional distress, you want relief immediately. And you will get it in a reasonable period of time only when the carbohydrate contains little or no fat.

LOSE STRESS WHILE LOSING WEIGHT

We believe that dieters – and everyone else – should eat to decrease feelings of stress because it is the natural thing to do.

We also believe that a diet should never eliminate those foods that decrease your feelings of stress. The Good Mood Diet ensures that your serotonin reserves are sufficient so those emotional events do not force you to overeat.

Because your serotonin levels will be constantly elevated, you will be buffered against any stresses that reoccur. You will not find yourself being upset by all the same things that bothered you before going on the diet.

That's what happened to Sandra, the overworked business executive who did not want to give up her night-time snacking but desperately needed to lose weight. Knee surgery had to wait until she lost over 13 kg (30 lb). Reluctantly, she agreed to go on the Good Mood Diet, but she was sure it would not help her relax in the evening.

Yet Sandra came back to us a week later a changed woman. 'Are you sure there were no tranquillizers in those crackers?' she asked. 'I was so laid back I even called my sister-in-law, who is always going on about my weight, to say hello. Normally, a conversation with her after a day at work makes me want to wolf down a large bag of crisps with dip. But I just let her words wash over me. Afterwards all my junk food went into the garbage bin. Now I feel calm and in control, from morning through to night.'

Serotonin turns off your appetite and turns on your good mood. Other diets cause stress. The Good Mood Diet, because it values carbohydrates, relieves stress.

ANTIDEPRESSANTS, WEIGHT GAIN AND THE SEROTONIN CONNECTION

Many people who gain weight on antidepressants decide to go on a low- or no-carbohydrate diet because overeating carbohydrates makes them gain weight. It seems like a logical approach, but it is misguided. Carbohydrate craving develops because the medications somehow cause the brain to need more serotonin. Eliminating or reducing carbohydrates to lose weight will only worsen the problem.

So far there is only one remedy for the unwanted side effect: the brain must produce additional serotonin.

That solution also has a scientific basis.

Many of the clients at the weight-loss clinic were people who had unexpectedly gained weight because they took antidepressants and mood stabilizers.

At the time Judy started the clinic, weight gain from antidepressant use was not well known. It was believed that the then-new class of antidepressants known as the SSRIs (selective serotonin reuptake inhibitors) did not cause weight gain. When Prozac first appeared, it caused some patients to lose weight during the first several weeks of treatment. But now it is known that after a few months on these drugs, weight increase can occur – usually about 6.8 to 16 kg (15 to 35 lb), though some people put on even more.[9–12]

No one really understands how antidepressants and mood stabilizers lead to increased appetite or, for that matter, fatigue. In fact, since these drugs act as an important therapy for mood disorders by prolonging the activity of serotonin, it is hard to understand how they can interfere with another serotonin activity, regulating appetite.

But they do interfere, and that is a major problem.

According to the Mental Health Foundation, at some point in their lives one in four women and one in ten men in the UK will suffer a period of depression serious enough to require treatment. The figures are similar in many other countries. And in the majority of cases the treatment prescribed will be a course of antidepressants.

Millions of people who are on antidepressants or mood regulators might be susceptible to the weight-gain side effect. The problem is serious enough for some patients to consider going off their medications to lose weight. This would be a mistake, particularly when these medications are effective.

Though our clients on medication had eating behaviours that were similar to those of our other clients, our clients on antidepressants showed specific additional symptoms that contributed to their weight gain.

They often felt thirsty because the medications left them with a dry mouth. Many satisfied their thirst with calorie-containing fizzy drinks and juices since they were unaware of how many extra calories they consumed each day in these drinks.

Others experienced dizziness or enormous fatigue, and some slept excessively. They often expressed the desire to be active but felt too tired to exercise.

And unlike the typical client, many of these people had never had a weight problem before they started on medication.

Claire was a typical client who thought she would never be able to take off the weight she had gained while taking an antidepressant following the death of her father. A professional violinist, she came to see us when she noticed that the skirts she had worn for performances for 15 years were too tight. 'I don't know what happened to me,' she stated. 'I'm 42 and I've been wearing size 10 since my school days. Now nothing fits.'

Before starting on the antidepressant, she had rarely snacked. 'I used to look down on my sister because she was always sneaking snacks between meals. Now I feel the need to eat constantly. I have my usual salad at lunch with a diet soft drink and an hour later, I'm roaming around the kitchen eating the kids' biscuits.'

Evenings were worse. 'It's a good thing I practise at night and my hands are busy. Otherwise I would be like a balloon.' She said she craved only junk food. 'My head keeps telling me to eat crunchy snack foods. I have probably consumed more crisps in the last 6 months than I have in the last 30 years.'

She was very sceptical that the Good Mood Diet would help, but she was willing to try since nothing else had worked. In a month, she had lost 2.7 kg (6 lb), and by the end of our programme she lost another 3.6 kg (8 lb). Along with losing weight, she finally lost her cravings and was back to eating normally.

After a few years of using the Good Mood Diet to help people lose weight, we compared the weight loss of people who were not on medications with those who were while they were on our programme. We found no difference in weight loss between the two groups, even though the medicated group was still on the drugs that had caused their weight gain in the first place.[12]

THE DIET THAT WORKS

The Good Mood Diet has three phases.

Serotonin Surge, phase 1, lasts for 2 weeks during which you'll eat three serotonin-boosting, high-carbohydrate, low-protein, low-fat snacks, along with three meals, every day. This frequent carbohydrate snacking will activate your brain's appetite- and mood-control systems as quickly as possible. Because evenings typically represent times when many people find it is hard to control overeating, you will increase serotonin production by eating a mainly carbohydrate dinner and enjoying a mid-evening snack.

Serotonin Balance, phase 2, lasts for 6 weeks. You will reduce your snacks to twice a day, one before lunch and the second late in the afternoon. Breakfast is the same as it was in the Serotonin Surge phase. At lunch, however, you will eat a little less protein, and you will add a little more protein to your dinner meal.

Serotonin Control, the 3rd phase, lasts for 4 weeks, though it can be followed for as long as you wish to lose weight. Breakfast remains the same. Lunch and dinner contain the same amounts of protein and carbohydrates as they did in the Serotonin Balance phase. Now, however,

---

Note: If you have diabetes or any medical condition that requires you to monitor what you eat, consult with your doctor before beginning the diet, and follow it under your doctor's guidance.

---

you will have one snack each day, late in the afternoon. The amount of the snack will be smaller, but you will be allowed to choose from a larger variety of snack foods (see page 66). To get you going, in the next chapter you'll identify all your personal eating triggers and discover the crucial difference between appetite and hunger.

Appetite, Hunger and Eating Triggers

Neither of us has ever encountered a client who claimed that hunger caused her or him to gain weight. And no one has ever told us that he or she stopped a diet because of unbearable hunger.

Virtually all of our clients gained weight or had trouble losing weight because they continued to eat after their bodies stopped being hungry. Often they ate so quickly that their stomachs filled up before their brains knew they had eaten anything. They stopped only when their stomachs felt sufficiently stuffed, when eating more became uncomfortable. Eventually, after the food was digested and their brains became aware of how much had been eaten, they would realize that they had eaten much too much. But by then, it was too late.

Like the rest of us, they often ate for reasons that had nothing to do with hunger. (How many times have you said you were not hungry before dessert and then just had to taste the luscious-looking cake or pastry?) The most common reasons our clients (and the rest of us) overeat have more to do with an automatic response to feeling bad, feeling stressed, or not knowing what to do next.

When people applied for research studies on obesity that were carried out at the Massachusetts Institute of Technology (MIT), they were given a questionnaire that asked why they thought they overate. The most common answers were:

- Because food was available
- For entertainment or distraction

- Because the clock said it was mealtime

- To join others who were eating something that looked appetizing

- Because they were bored, tired, restless or annoyed or there was nothing good on television

- Because it was the only good thing they could do for themselves that day

This type of eating has nothing to do with hunger, but it has everything to do with how important food is in our emotional lives.

Recently, another important reason for overeating was discovered: being on medications, such as antidepressants, that block the brain's ability to turn off appetite.

The problem our clients faced was that all the diets they had been on previously focused only on controlling hunger – not on satisfying the urge to eat that can arise when a person is not feeling hungry.

Karen, a young woman who wanted to lose 35 kg (5½ st), struggled with this problem. She could not remember ever being hungry, even as a child. That wasn't surprising, because her mother was always ready to feed her between meals, after meals – whenever she was not eating. And Karen continued to feed herself the same way as an adult.

'I don't know what it's like to feel that I have to eat immediately because I'm starved,' she said. 'Real hunger? What's that?'

HUNGER IS NOT WHAT YOU MIGHT THINK IT IS

Consider this: if you ate only when you were really hungry and then only enough food to ease that hunger, it's unlikely that you would ever have a weight problem.

Additionally, if you ate solely in response to your body's need for fuel, you would be satisfied with anything that met your body's demands for calories.

It's also not unusual to feel hunger sensations during the first few days of a diet, especially if the plan is extremely low in calories. Yet many people claim that after a week or so, their hunger goes away. We have talked to people on 500-calorie-a-day liquid diets who were able to stay on such a restricted regime for weeks. For them, hunger was not an issue because their bodies had adjusted to taking in fewer calories.

The same lack of hunger is typical of people who have gone through surgical procedures to reduce the size of their stomachs. They may eat only tiny amounts of food at any time and claim never to be hungry.

What is so interesting is that once people on low-calorie liquid diets are allowed to eat a wider variety of foods, they often find themselves eating more than their bodies need. They eat out of appetite, not hunger. The same may happen with those who have had their stomachs reduced via surgery, but the consequences of eating more can make them ill.

What we are talking about here is appetite, not hunger.

APPETITE VERSUS HUNGER

Do you eat because of hunger? Or do you eat because of appetite? There is a big difference.

When you eat to satisfy hunger, you might enjoy the seasoning, taste, texture or colour of the food. But your primary reason for eating is to nourish your body. Once you eat enough to satisfy your nutritional needs, you stop.

However, when you eat to satisfy your appetite, hunger may not be as important as other stimuli. These include your mood, a craving for a particular food, social cues, the pleasure of eating, habit or food availability. These appetite signals, rather than hunger, lead to eating more calories than your body needs, and as a result, you gain weight or cannot lose excess weight.

Here is a simple way to determine if your appetite, rather than your hunger, affects what you eat. Do you ever:

- Plan on ordering just a cup of coffee but add a pastry or a slice of cake because it looks so tempting?

- See someone on the street eating an ice cream cone and decide you must also have one, right now?

- Spend inordinate amounts of time ordering from a menu because you can't decide what you feel like eating?

- Find yourself ordering doughnuts or other fried foods at a fair because the smell is so enticing?

- Have no intention of ordering anything else – until you see the desserts on offer?

- Feel you have to sample everything at a buffet no matter how full you are?

- Find it impossible to resist helping yourself to the biscuits or other snacks in the kitchen at work?

- Eat the crisps that come with a sandwich even though you did not order them?

If you answered yes to any of these questions, your appetite has controlled what you eat.

But remember, there is nothing wrong with your appetite helping you make food choices, as long as it does not lead you to continue eating after you stop being hungry. Appetite makes certain that foods give you pleasure.

With our clients we have found that, generally, as the day progresses, appetite plays a more important role in what, how much, and when they eat. For example, a number of our clients choose the same breakfast every day, the same breakfast they have been eating for years. The meal satisfies their hunger. Lunch is often a meal squeezed in between work, family and household obligations. But later in the day, factors such as stress, boredom, social interaction, loneliness, entitlement to eat and brain chemistry may cause appetite, not hunger, to influence when and what food is eaten.

Appetite, when uncontrolled, leads you to consume unneeded calories – a major obstacle to losing weight and keeping it off.

The first step to losing weight and keeping it off is to become aware of when your desire to eat is generated by the untimely urges of appetite. The next step is to feed your body the carbohydrates it craves so the brain can produce serotonin and thereby curb that appetite.

THE BRAIN, APPETITE AND CARBOHYDRATE CRAVING

Pressures on appetite, including the sight, smell and availability of food, are normally to be found everywhere, and they're compounded when you're on a high-protein, low-carbohydrate diet; taking antidepressant medication; or using food to alter your mood. No matter what the cause, the result may be that you have a lot of trouble controlling what and how much food you eat.

While you probably can employ willpower to turn away from fried fish or barbecued pork ribs, you may be powerless to resist baked goods, pasta and their carb cousins. The reason for this specific, very tough-to-ignore craving for carbohydrates is that your brain is forcing you to yearn for them so that it can produce serotonin.

TEST YOURSELF

Take a minute to answer the questions in the self-tests that follow to see which of these brain-based appetite triggers is affecting your eating. Questionnaires similar to these have been used in our research studies and our clinical practice.

You may believe that you already know what is causing your appetite disturbance, but taking the tests is worthwhile anyway. You may find that more than one trigger is causing problems with your eating control.

That's what happened to Peter, a 47-year-old executive whose doctor suggested that he try our diet plan. During a brief consultation, he told us he knew why he had gained 16 kg (2½ st). It was a side effect of his antidepressant.

'Just tell me what to eat,' he insisted. 'I don't need to discuss anything else.'

Initially, we complied with his request. But after a few weeks, Peter admitted that he was having trouble staying on the diet and returned to find out what else might be affecting his eating. As it happened, he was also eating due to emotional distress.

The eldest son of five children, he was shouldering the entire responsibility for taking care of his father, who was in a nursing home, and his mother, who had recently suffered a stroke. Despite being very angry at his siblings' lack of accountability, he still could not bring himself to criticize them directly. Instead, he used food to quiet his anger and help him remain calm when he visited his parents or planned to speak with his brothers and sisters.

Similarly, our client Deirdre had multiple reasons for overeating. Deirdre was 27 when antidepressant medication led to a weight gain of nearly 9 kg (1½ st). 'I wanted to get rid of the pounds and did what everyone else was doing: a low-carb, high-protein diet,' she told us. 'But it backfired. The lack of carbohydrates on the diet just intensified the cravings caused by my medication. After I was on the diet for a couple of weeks, I would wake up at night to eat. After a while I gave up and kept cookies on my bedside table. When I woke up I reached for a handful, even before I got out of bed.'

Section A: High-Protein Weight-Loss Diets and Your Brain

Circle yes or no to answer each question. If you haven't used one of these diets recently, skip to Section B on page 29.

If you've been on this kind of diet recently, has it made you:

Obsess about eating sweet or starchy snacks?	Yes	No
Feel drained and without energy?	Yes	No
Jumpy and unable to concentrate?	Yes	No
Moody and prone to grumpiness?	Yes	No
Sleep badly or wake up frequently?	Yes	No
Less able to handle stress?	Yes	No
Feel full but not satisfied?	Yes	No
Get angry easily?	Yes	No

If you answered yes to four or more of the eight questions, your diet may have affected the serotonin level in your brain. It's no secret that food plans with too little carbohydrate can have a negative effect on the serotonin level. Uncontrollable carbohydrate cravings and a bad mood are the consequences.

After a few days of feeding your brain the carbs it needs, enough new serotonin is produced to restore your control over eating. When that happens, the cravings for carbohydrates begin to diminish, as does the desire to overeat.

If your answers indicate that a high-protein diet has altered your mood and appetite control, the first part of the diet plan, the Serotonin Surge phase, will quickly reinforce your control over your eating and most likely restore your good mood. And it will do both of these things while you lose weight.

Section B: Emotions and Your Brain

Circle yes or no to answer each question.

Are you someone who reaches for foods containing sugar, starch or both when:

You are bored, tired or lonely?	Yes	No
You are angry, irritated, tense or anxious?	Yes	No
You are trying to deal with a stressful situation?	Yes	No
You feel in need of a reward, distraction or relaxation?	Yes	No
You want to delay doing something?	Yes	No
You are trying to relax so you can fall asleep?	Yes	No
You don't know what to do next?	Yes	No
It is time to eat, because eating time is the only time you allow yourself to relax?	Yes	No
The dark days of autumn and winter cause you to feel down in the dumps, very tired, and cause you to crave sweets?	Yes	No
You feel edgy or depressed because you just stopped smoking?	Yes	No

Additional questions for women:

It is a few days before your period and you are experiencing PMS mood swings?	Yes	No
Menopausal changes in hormones make you exhausted, depressed or anxious?	Yes	No

If you answered yes to four or more of the questions, you are one of many people who eat as a way of making yourself feel better or, at least, less bad. If this is the case, recognize that your brain responds positively to your eating. When you reach for carbohydrates to soothe yourself, you are eating those foods because they will improve your mood. Your frame of mind brightens, even if it's just a little, because of the increase in serotonin.

At some point in your life you learned, perhaps subconsciously, that after you ate you could better endure your problems. So if your motto is 'I am upset, therefore I will eat something sweet or starchy,' you are fortunate (although it may not seem that way right now). Nature has given you an effective and easy way to make yourself feel better when there is no other way of dealing with stress except to cope. By choosing foods that will increase serotonin production, relief will be on the way.

But, you might be saying, how can I lose weight and overeat carbs the way I have been when I am upset?

You can't. The calorie content of the foods you have been eating is too high to allow you to lose weight and keep it off. You probably were eating larger amounts of carbohydrates than you needed to make serotonin. But, as you will see in Chapters 5 and 6, you will be able to eat many emotionally soothing and delicious foods at mealtimes and as snacks. They will satisfy your cravings and help to relieve stress. Their controlled calorie content will promote, not prevent, weight loss.

That's what Janet discovered when she came to see us for a consultation. She was not sure she wanted to enter our weight-loss programme. 'Everyone tells me that the only way I am going to lose weight is to stop eating carbohydrates,' the 41-year-old stated, 'so I really don't think your diet plan is right for me. But on the other hand, every time I stop eating carbohydrates, I become really upset, anxious and nasty to be with. The diets become intolerable.'

Janet, who had gained over 20 kg (3 st) over 2 years, had numerous emotionally driven reasons to overeat. She worked 14-hour days because her office was understaffed. After several disastrous relationships, her social life had stalled. Her family nagged her incessantly about losing weight. A beloved cat she had had for 15 years had died. In response to all of these events, she ate and ate.

We explained that the carbohydrates she would be eating at specific times of the day would help to buffer her against distress. But we also warned her that food was not going to solve any of her problems. With our help and that of a therapist, she eventually overcame the problems and lost the extra weight. And it stayed off.

New stresses replaced the old ones, but as Janet told us, 'Now when I'm upset, I know what carbohydrates to eat. Once they calm me down, I can figure out what to do about my problems – or even do nothing about them. At least I'm not eating my way through my troubles anymore.'

Section C: Antidepressants and Your Brain

Circle yes or no to answer each question. If you are not on antidepressants or any related medication, skip this section.

If you have been on an antidepressant medication for longer than 3 or 4 weeks, has it made you:

Increase your consumption of sweet or starchy carbohydrates (in meals or as snacks) instead of protein and vegetables?	Yes No
Eat more than you did before starting the medication?	Yes No
Think about eating all the time, even after finishing a meal?	Yes No
Feel like eating late at night or wake up at night wanting to eat?	Yes No
Have an uncontrollable craving for sweet and starchy foods?	Yes No
Feel more fatigued than you did before taking the medication?	Yes No
Gain weight?	Yes No

If you answered 'yes' to four or more of the seven questions, you may be experiencing antidepressant-induced carbohydrate cravings. After several weeks of use, many people begin having a constant craving for carbohydrates.

Audrey's comments are typical of those we've heard from people who experienced medication-induced weight gain.

'I never ate junk food until 6 months ago, when I started taking medication for my depression,' the 30-ish woman explained. 'In college, I used to feel superior to my friends who lived on chocolate and chips. I was the health-food queen, a regular at the salad bar. Now I can't stop myself from gorging on cakes. I've put on 16 kg (2½ st) – and the cravings won't stop.'

The powerful urge to eat carbohydrates, the feeling of never being satisfied and the need to eat more are all common side effects of antidepressants. It is hard to know who is bothered more by this: people who were always thin and now are heavy, or people who always had a weight problem that has gotten worse. It is a bad situation for anyone who is affected.

We found that when clients come to consult with us because of antidepressant-related weight gain, they are either consuming the wrong kind of carbohydrates or eating them at the wrong time. Most of them tend to eat their carbs as dessert or start snacking soon after a meal is finished.

What they don't realize is that part of the problem is timing. Their carbohydrate intake coincides with protein digestion. The protein interferes with the ability of the carbohydrates to start the serotonin-making process.

Additionally, many exacerbate their weight-gain problem by choosing snacks so high in calories and fat that their daily calorie intake becomes excessive. Many of our clients never notice how many calories a chocolate bar or a pastry contains.

Fortunately, it's not necessary to stop taking your antidepressant to lose weight. We were able to help people lose weight on our diet plan even though they were still on the same type and dosage of medication that had caused their weight gain to begin with.

Nonetheless, you should be aware that the weight might not come off as easily as removing a jacket. Losing this weight requires that you establish healthy eating and exercise patterns. You must start exercising, even though the thought of doing so with the extra weight may make you reluctant to do so. (If you have drug-related fatigue, see Chapter 7 for suggestions on how to start slowly and build up stamina.)

Recently we saw a school nurse who had always been the right weight for her height. When she was treated for depression with an antidepressant following her husband's death, she found herself gaining weight. Admitting that she was very aware of her changed eating habits and lack of exercise, she told us, 'Before, I always ate a piece of fruit for an afternoon snack. Sweets never appealed to me. But now I eat chocolate every afternoon and pastries from a local bakery after supper.

'I used to walk at least 3 miles every day. Now if I walk half a mile it's unusual. I feel like a thin person stuck in a fat body and I don't know how to get out.'

But in less than 4 months on the Good Mood Diet she was able to get out of that body and return to being a thin person. Once her cravings were controllable, her food choices reverted back to those of her pre-medication days and she was motivated to exercise. Her stamina quickly returned. Even though she sometimes was tired and didn't really feel like exercising, knowing that she could walk the way she had in the past was enough to keep her moving.

FREQUENTLY ASKED QUESTIONS

Why does my antidepressant medication help my mood but not my appetite? Isn't all serotonin the same?

Even though all serotonin is the same, serotonin plays many roles in the brain. One role is to keep your mood stable and regulated. Another role is to regulate your appetite. We don't understand how an antidepressant medication that helps serotonin improve mood and take away depression can interfere with serotonin's role in appetite control. But the unhappy fact is that most antidepressants may cause weight gain. The happy fact is that the Good Mood Diet will make you lose the weight.

Won't my brain be making too much serotonin if I eat all those carbohydrates, therefore affecting my medication?

No, eating carbohydrates will not make your medication less effective. Since serotonin may be affecting certain aspects of your mood not influenced by antidepressants, like grumpiness or impatience, you may find yourself in an all-around better mood. None of our clients has experienced negative effects from producing more serotonin. No one has had to adjust his or her dosage of antidepressants because of eating more potatoes or pasta.

How can you suggest eating as a way of solving problems? It seems like an easy way out.

Eating is never the way to solve problems. But you need to be calm and composed to deal with your problems. We believe that if you can increase serotonin by eating carbohydrates, you will be in the right frame of mind to deal with stress. Food never removes problems.

Why has everyone told me to stop eating carbohydrates so that I can be thin?

People who gave you that advice didn't understand that you can eat to make yourself feel better – and that there's nothing wrong with this approach. Nature has given us an effective way of improving our mood. When this was discovered at MIT, people understood that they could use carbohydrates – in the right amounts and at the right times – to make themselves feel good and lose weight. When carbohydrates were removed from the diet, the drop in serotonin made people lose their good mood and their ability to control their appetite. That is a high price to pay for losing a little weight.

CHAPTER THREE

If You Want to Change Your Weight, You Have to Change Your Mind, Too

Now you know why you overeat. It may be due to antidepressants, a dietary imbalance, or emotional causes. Once and for all, you want to take control of that overeating, to make a change for your physical well-being, your looks or the way you feel about yourself.

Losing weight and keeping it off requires more than changing the way you eat and exercise. It demands a change of mind, a commitment to becoming and staying a thinner, fitter and more energized you.

And that requires facing and overcoming the biggest obstacle to weight loss – life.

LIFE TENDS TO GET IN THE WAY

No matter how much the Good Mood Diet controls your food choices, you still must face day-to-day obstacles that threaten to derail the best intentions.

Temptations lurk everywhere: in your kitchen, in your workplace, along the streets and in the supermarket. That's why dieters are so successful when they retreat to spas or residential diet centres, where all the temptations are removed.

Nancy, a client who had been on every diet known to the Western world, told us that she was successful in losing weight when she took a 6-month leave of absence from her job. She did nothing but go to diet meetings and the gym and cook the foods she was allowed to eat.

'My social life was non-existent and I refused to go to my friends' and relatives' homes to eat. I became a recluse, but a thin one. Of course, when I went back to work and faced the world again, the weight came back in a few weeks.'

Nancy's post-recluse experience mirrors that of many us.

Consider just a few of the endless opportunities that could prompt you to deviate from the Good Mood Diet. Going to a restaurant and selecting a dish that does not conform to the guidelines of the plan, eating a little more than the recommended portion size and simply judging the amount you think you should eat rather than measuring it are just a few. Then there is the choice of lying on the sofa and watching TV or walking on the treadmill.

You must believe that you will succeed in losing weight. That's why changing your mind is so important. We strongly believe that successful weight loss hinges on a mental shift acknowledging that what you are committed to doing is possible, even with all those pitfalls along the way. Doing so practically guarantees weight loss.

The decisions to stick to the diet or deviate will never disappear. Should you eat those biscuits in the office kitchen rather than the permitted snack? Should you walk or take the car? Can you order a speciality coffee with whipped cream or must you settle for coffee with skimmed milk and non-calorie sweetener? Should you order what looks good or what is good for your diet?

You've made a commitment to lose weight, and we are going to help you stick with it. Here are some simple suggestions to get you over the hurdles that are sure to block your way. They work for our clients. They will work for you, too.

A WEEK OF FOOD TEMPTATIONS

Let's follow Mary, a 36-year-old primary school teacher. At our request, she wrote down the temptations she faced during 1 week as she fought the battle of 'to eat or not to eat'.

Monday, the First Skirmish: The Coffee Shop

What I thought I wanted. 'I was waiting my turn in the coffee shop for the coffee I drink on the way to work. I found myself staring at the trays of iced doughnuts, muffins and bagels and thinking that eating a buttered blueberry muffin along with my coffee would get the day off to a perfect start.'

What I did. 'I remembered that not 45 minutes before I had eaten my bran flakes, strawberries and skimmed milk. Was I really hungry for another breakfast? No, I wasn't. It was my appetite talking. Besides, I knew that there were snacks in my bag for me to eat later. I ordered my coffee – and nothing else.'

Tuesday, the Second Attack: The Birthday Party

What I thought I wanted. 'My class has nearly 30 kids in it, and birthday parties, along with holiday events, are part of the school calendar. Today was Jenny's birthday, and her mother delivered a tray of beautifully decorated cakes, with one for each child and one for me, too. Now these weren't ordinary homemade cakes because Jenny's mother is an excellent baker. Her son was in my class 2 years ago, so I know. Those minicakes are cream-filled and iced with thick frosting. They are so delicious and so hard to resist.'

What I did. 'Before she left, I thanked Jenny's mother and told her that I wanted to 'save mine for later'. I glanced at that cake and then focused on the wall clock for 20 seconds. Then I asked myself if I would really miss the treat if I didn't eat it. After all, there were many other celebrations to come (and I could deal with them when they arrived). I took the cake to the teacher's room and left it on the plate with the other treats that appear there daily. Then it was time to enjoy my own snack, which was sweet and satisfying, and no one was the wiser, except for me. There was an extra benefit for my students: I could concentrate on them and not on food.'

Wednesday, the Third Clash: The Supermarket

What I thought I wanted. 'Okay, maybe I like to torture myself, but I love food shopping at my local supermarket. It is gigantic and almost every aisle has a place where someone gives out free food samples.

Nibbling on the cheese cubes, little cups of lasagne or chilli, or choco-late chip cookies makes food shopping fun.

'Of course, I would usually pick up an extra few hundred calories along with my shopping by the time I exited the store. Today the sam-ples were really torturous: two new flavours of a premium ice cream that I really love plus a different kind of potato crisp.'

What I did. 'Before I went into the supermarket I ate my afternoon snack in the car while I listened to part of a CD I really like. It was my private mini-break, just for me. By the time I went food shopping, I was mellow and not interested in eating. I bought what I needed and cruised right by the samples.'

Thursday: The Home Front

What I thought I wanted. 'My husband isn't on the diet with me, and he insists on a big meal at the end of the day, which means a large slab of protein on a plate. Once the weather turns warm, he goes into cave-man mode, fires up the barbecue, and cooks himself steak or hamburg-ers or chicken. Everything smells divine, plus the aromas remind me of camping trips when I was growing up. The gravitational pull of meat sizzling over coals is really powerful.'

What I did. 'I did taste what my husband prepared for himself and then I ate what I had planned for myself. But here's the thing: I saved a portion of meat, sliced it thin and marinated it. I planned to eat it, along with some of the leftover grilled vegetables, for lunch the next day. There's a lot to be said for delayed gratification, because I will be looking forward to my lunch as a special treat. Plus I got to eat a lot of carbs for dinner, something I never thought I would be able to do on any diet.'

Friday: The Reward

What I thought I wanted. 'When the kids leave on Friday afternoon, I feel entitled to a reward. I made it through another week of 10-year-olds. Usually I go out to a local pizza place with a couple of my teacher friends and we share an 'end of the week' pizza and, once in a while, a pitcher of beer. We gossip, exchange funny stories about what went on in school, and eat.

What I did. 'I knew that the afternoon pizza and my diet were incompatible. So I convinced my friends to come with me to a knit-ting shop that opened a few minutes away. The owner gives free lessons to groups of three or more. They loved the idea, and I brought snacks for all of us to eat while we were looking through the wool. It was great fun and we decided to go every Friday rather than eating pizza.'

Saturday: Shopping Day

What I thought I wanted. 'Saturday is shopping day. I come from a large family and someone is always celebrating a birthday or graduating or getting married. So I shop for lots of gifts. This activity also gives me an excuse to go to the food court in the shopping centre, which I love. I always want to eat something from all the concessions. Sometimes I choose something from each of my four favourite concessions and if I am really feeling indulgent, I finish with a small sundae.'

What I did. 'When I entered the food court, I walked around to all the different counters, looking at everything but not ordering. It was sort of like window-shopping. I knew that I could afford only a certain number of calories, just as I can only afford to buy certain articles of clothing. I decided to use the same technique I use when shopping for clothing or shoes to keep myself from making an impulsive purchase. I discovered that one restaurant had great salads with grilled chicken and low-fat salad dressing and ordered that for lunch. It tasted really good. Of course I also gave myself credit for remembering to eat my pre-lunch snack while I was still shopping. It curbed my appetite, just as I knew it would.'

Sunday: The Church Social Hour

What I thought I wanted. 'I sing in my church choir on Sundays and because I have to be in church by 8:30 a.m., I eat breakfast really early. Right after the morning service ends there is always a spread in the social hall featuring coffee, tea and lots of cakes. I am ashamed to say that I usually eat more than my share because by then I am starved. I probably eat the equivalent of two lunches in cakes.'

What I did. 'I brought my own snack and I started to eat it while I was taking off my choir robe. I took the rest downstairs with me to the social hall and ate it with a cup of coffee. It helped not to go near the tables with all the goodies, so I stayed on the other side of the room and chatted with people. By the time I finished my snack, the table looked as if locusts had descended on it – really unappealing. I was really proud of myself. Looking back on the week, I realized that it wasn't that hard to win these eating battles. It just took a little thought, a little willpower and a little carbohydrate.'

THE SEVEN MENTAL STRATEGIES THAT WON THE DAY

Mary utilized a simple set of skills.

Look before you eat. Unless Mary decided to skip her early morning coffee spot, and every other breakfast place, she was going to be faced with a tantalizing selection of baked goods. Shops fill display cases for a good reason; presenting their offerings attracts buyers. (Ask yourself: If I didn't see that almond croissant, would I want one?) If you're not truly hungry, realize that you don't want, or need, the extra calories. Focus on the difference between appetite and hunger.

Practise the 20-second rule. There it was, the ideal cake, and it had her name on it. Nonetheless, Mary applied the 20-second rule. She regarded her potential downfall briefly and then switched her focus for a short time. Give yourself 20 seconds to consider whether you really want to squander calories on a piece of cake.

Be responsible for what you eat. Mary was accountable for her food intake. At dinner she made decisions that were in her favour, both at that moment and for the next day. She was in control and she felt good about it. Plus, she wasn't suffering from pangs of deprivation or feelings of being left out. Take charge of your calories, your weight loss, and, most of all, yourself.

Snack before you food shop. Mary knew that having her serotonin-boosting snack before going into the supermarket would help her control her habitual free-sample tasting. Take the time to enjoy your snacks as well as the calm and relaxed feeling they give.

Give yourself the gift of fun, not food. Mary found that an end-of-the-school-week treat did not have to be either high calorie or fat filled. She identified something else that would be fun to do (and even brought snacks). Be aware that there are lots of treats that not only satisfy but also help you lose weight.

Window-shop for food. There is no avoiding the overabundance of food available for the asking. Bakeries often place small samples of goodies on the counter for tasting. Up-market chocolate shops will provide tiny tastes. Sometimes it is hard to avoid being tempted to eat when you see other people around you biting into their almond croissants or double choc-chip cookies.

Live within your calorie budget and 'shop' for the best calorie values. Assess whether or not being attracted to foods means that you really want them.

Know your enemy. Mary was finally able to stop her hungry assault on the after-church goodies by acknowledging their tempting presence and providing her private defence weapon – her own snack. Moreover, she did something else very effectively. She busied herself by talking to her friends, and that kept her away from the treat-laden table.

It is possible to face, and conquer, your food temptations.

But what about the other daily stresses that can undermine the most committed dieter?

STRESS HAPPENS

Stress hits on a continual basis. Most stressors cannot be ignored or wished away. Even with the soothing effects of serotonin, you will still find yourself affected by those negative daily events. A breakdown on the public transport system, a traffic jam, teenagers (need we say more?), too little sleep, unexpected bills, too much to do, too little time to do it, sickness, bad news, trouble with a boyfriend or girlfriend, family dynamics – the list goes on.

While there often isn't much you can do to change these exterior circumstances, you can alter your interior circumstances. That is, you can take quick steps to de-stress yourself. A mental break will make you feel better. And when you feel better you are less apt to be tempted to eat.

The next time stress pushes you, push back with these mini-breaks. Think you're too busy? They require only 2 to 5 minutes. Surely you can spare that much for your peace of mind.

■ Do a 1- or 2-minute meditation. Close your eyes and clear your mind. To give yourself some mental space, don't make judgements about or react to the thoughts that come into your head. For example, if a thought like 'This job is driving me crazy' or 'If he doesn't get off that mobile phone in 5 seconds I'm going to explode' crosses your mind, let it go.

■ Sit down and read the newspaper, a magazine article or a few pages of a book for 2 minutes.

■ Listen to 5 minutes of soothing music.

■ Tune in to a daytime TV talk show. Five minutes of viewing will reassure you that your problems are not so bad.

■ Turn to the sports section and either bemoan or cheer your team of choice.

■ Gaze out a window and allow yourself to daydream for a couple of minutes.

■ Keep a snow globe on your desk. Whenever you feel stressed, grab it, shake it a few times, and watch the flakes fly.

■ If you don't have pets or are too far away from them to have their influence magically lower your blood pressure, buy a goldfish and keep the tank near your workspace. A few minutes of watching it swim is amazingly hypnotic.

You can avoid some stresses with a little pre-planning and anticipation. No surprises means decreased stress levels. All kinds of stresses can be reduced. Consider:

The 'no time for anything' stress When this happens there is one thing to do: ask for help. At home, can't your family contribute 20 minutes to helping you with the washing, preparing lunches, going to the supermarket, emptying the dishwasher, making beds, or cleaning out the cat's litter tray?

At your job, if work is being piled on you and the only way you can handle it is to work late and on weekends, and if this is making it impossible for you to eat and exercise healthily, then you need to do something about it. Unless working 80 hours a week was in your job description, you are sacrificing your health for your job.

One client, a young lawyer, often stayed in the office all evening to do her assigned work. Consequently, she gained more than 18 kg (2 st 9 lb) over the first 18 months of her job. She never arrived at home before 8 or 9 at night and she usually worked Saturdays. There was little time to take care of basic needs such as going food shopping and doing housework, much less getting adequate sleep or enjoying a social life. In discussing her work situation, we discovered

SEROTONIN: THE STRESS REDUCER

Carbohydrates function as the buffer between you and whatever bothers you. By making enough serotonin to keep you calm and able to cope, carbohydrates act like a bandage that goes over a wound and keeps it clean and safe while it heals. And just as a bandage has no effect on what caused the wound, eating will never affect the cause of the stress. But because carbohydrates help to render the problems bearable, you will have the time and energy to try to figure out ways of decreasing these problems or making them less important.

That's why the Good Mood Diet plan is different from other programmes. The food choices it provides are powerful weapons at your disposal. Instead of falling victim to your appetite, you will curb it, forget about it, and go about your business.

Knowing you can control your eating can free you to take care of yourself in other important ways.

You can use food as a dependable ally. Rather than letting your appetite spin out of control, which will only add extra weight and more stress, you can take charge. As soon as you feel, or anticipate, a stressful moment arriving, you will be ready to deal with it.

Is anything more stress reducing than that?

that every lawyer in the firm dumped work on her because she was at the bottom of the pecking order. We encouraged her to go to the manager of the firm and discuss whether she was supposed to handle so much. When she did so, the manager, appalled, immediately decreased her workload.

The '4:30 in the afternoon, home with the kids and preparing dinner' stress The kids are underfoot, your patience is on a short leash, and you are in the kitchen. This is a recipe for overeating. How do you defuse this situation? Plan ahead.

If you have the option of spending 20 minutes in the morning doing some preparation for dinner, that will leave you less to do before you eat. If not, devote a couple of weekend hours to preparing food and freezing it.

Eat your snack before your cravings get the best of you. For example, if you automatically start to nibble around 4:30 p.m., have your snack about 45 minutes sooner. By 4:30, your appetite will be subdued so you can concentrate on other things, like preparing dinner or finishing up the day's work.

The 'dark and cold Sunday afternoon and I have nothing to do' stress Sundays come around once a week. Prepare ahead of time. By Tuesday, know what your Sunday afternoon options are. You can contribute your time and volunteer to help out at your local hospital or animal shelter.

The 'no time to food shop' stress Does your local supermarket have a food delivery service? You can order via computer and have food delivered. Or go to the supermarket early on a weekend morning, when stores are usually quiet and it takes much less time to get in and out. If you have the storage space, buy a month's supplies of storecupboard items at a time.

The 'everyone makes demands on me and I don't have any time for myself' stress The answer is simple – just say no. The first hundred times you do this you will probably feel guilty. Get over it. Instead, take pleasure in the thought that by saying no to others, you're saying yes to doing something for yourself – and you will be able to give your renewed self to others.

The 'only pleasure I have is eating' stress Come on. Admit it. There must be something you would love to do for fun. You did it in the past and you can do it again no matter how 'silly' it might seem now that you're all grown-up. One of our clients, a recently divorced young man, was totally resistant to our typical suggestions. When 'play the bagpipes' was suggested as a last resort his eyes lit up. 'Okay!' he exclaimed. 'I haven't played them for years. And they are still in my cupboard.'

The 'I am so tired from lack of sleep I have to eat' stress Too little sleep can have a big impact on your appetite. Eating is not a substitute for sleeping, and although eating will keep you awake, you (along with your diet) will benefit if you go to bed, rather than to the kitchen, when you are exhausted.

One client who stayed awake much too late at night was so exhausted during the day that she ate constantly to keep herself going. She hated getting ready for bed and would avoid cleaning her face, brushing her teeth and getting into her pyjamas until she was so tired that she would go to the kitchen and eat. By getting ready for bed by 9 p.m., she had no excuse to eat to stay awake.

Those of you on antidepressants and other medications that make you feel tired and sleep excessively must make sure that you put aside enough time to get the sleep your body and medication demands. Otherwise you will be especially vulnerable to eating out of exhaustion.

The 'diet is not working for me' stress Most of dieting is about changing your mind. Your old frame of mind pushes you to eat what you please and ignore whether you are exercising enough. We know that it is very challenging to change familiar and comfortable behaviours, even if you know you must. For some it may be as difficult as emigrating to a new country where the language, means of transportation, housing and customs are all different. But remember that every day, people leave places where they feel oppressed or uncomfortable even if they have known that place for a long time.

Finally, dieting should not add another stress to your life. Once you make the commitment to yourself, do what you must to make it easier for yourself. That may mean crossing something off your calendar. For instance, pick one lunch hour a week when you will exercise. Schedule no business lunches for that day. Or, instead of snacking while you answer all your e-mails at night, leave them and go to sleep. They will be waiting for you. And if you usually cook different dishes for each family member, pick one day each week when you all eat the same meal for dinner. Remember that you made a pledge to yourself. You owe it to yourself to make it happen.

If you find it extremely difficult to change your eating, exercise and social habits, ask yourself if you are really ready to change your mind.

READY, OR NOT

Our client Neil's story is a terrific example of knowing when you are ready to lose weight.

'Of course I want to lose weight, but I'm really busy' were his first words to us. A senior manager at a biotechnology start-up and the father of two children under the age of 10, Neil had gained 16 kg (2½ st) in the year since starting antidepressant medication. To his wife's dismay, every evening after a large supper he would wander in and out of the kitchen, alternating bowls of sweet cereal with scoops of ice cream topped with handfuls of nuts and mounds of whipped cream. Concerned that their valuable time together was being squandered, she recognized that his weight gain was a critical issue for both of them and convinced him to see us.

Tip: Weight loss is a lifetime commitment that plays out 1 day at a time.

From the beginning, it was clear that Neil was not motivated. He didn't follow the eating plan, he kept promising to go the gym in his office building but didn't, and he continued to put in long hours to keep up with his work demands. After a few weeks Neil finally told us what was readily apparent. 'I do feel guilty about not trying. But the truth is that I'm just not prepared to make the kind of commitment I need to in order to lose weight.'

Neil's honesty was a big step, and we told him that when he was ready he would be welcomed back.

Six months later Neil returned. He was ready to begin the diet plan and schedule exercise into his diary. Additionally, he decided to work fewer hours no matter how much he wanted to get done. Spending more time with his wife and kids became a priority. Eight months later he had lost 18 kg (2 st 9 lb), renewed his relationship with his family, and rediscovered himself in the process. 'I feel and look better at 43 than I did at 33. I guess I just had to wait until my mind was made up to change my body. I'm just sorry I waited so long to do it,' he said.

FREQUENTLY ASKED QUESTIONS

Do I really need a reason beyond the obvious one – I don't like being overweight – to motivate me to lose weight?

Yes, you do. Simply not wanting to be overweight is a wish, not a plan. Perhaps you can recognize how being overweight is an obstacle to achieving a more fulfilling life. Or that if you lose weight you will feel more empowered. One way to motivate yourself is to recognize how gratifying it is to make a commitment to a goal, identify the specific steps to get there, follow your plan, and reap the rewards. If you follow our plan, you will lose weight and feel better about yourself and your body.

I've made commitments before and dropped them. How can I stay committed to losing weight this time?

You must be realistic about the process and commit to only what will fit into your current lifestyle. Also, you must take responsibility for your decision to lose weight. Even though The Good Mood Diet will help control your appetite and boost your mood, you still need to be aware of what (and when) you eat and that you must exercise.

THE LAMEST EXCUSES NOT TO LOSE WEIGHT

Here are our all-time favourite excuses used by clients not to lose weight.

- I'm storing weight for winter.
- When I lose weight, my face gets too thin.
- I've got too much going on.
- This is the weight I'm supposed to be.
- My sibling/friend/spouse/relative will feel jealous.
- Someone has to eat the leftovers.
- I like my love handles. There is more of me to love.
- My metabolism is slow.
- Everyone else loses weight on diets, but I don't.
- There's nothing else to do but eat.
- My cholesterol and blood pressure are normal, so I have nothing to worry about.
- My husband and I are eating partners. If I go on a diet, he won't have anyone to eat with.
- My mother/spouse/friend will be mad at me.
- I have big bones.
- I paid for the food. I'm going to eat it.
- Nobody likes a 'loser'.

What can I do about people who don't support my efforts?

Responding to adversity is one of the best ways to strengthen your resolve. But it doesn't have to be a battle. If someone expects you to eat foods that are not part of your plan, there are polite ways to say, 'No, thank you'. Be sure to acknowledge and praise the efforts that may have gone into food preparation for a celebration or dinner with friends or family. Saying 'Thanks, I've had enough' can also help. Find someone from your family or set of friends and colleagues who will support your weight-loss efforts.

I used to be really fit and thin before I went on antidepressants. Now I weigh at least 13.5 kg [2 st] more than I should. Do you think I should stop taking the antidepressants to stay on the diet?

No. If you are to make any change in your medication, it must be done in consultation with your doctor and should be based on whether or not you need the medication and not simply on what you weigh. The plan will work whether or not you are on antidepressants. Our research shows that people on antidepressants lose weight as effectively as people who are not on these drugs.

How do I explain my snacking and the rest of the diet? I don't want to tell people I'm on yet another diet.

Reluctance to mention your dieting if you failed in the past is understandable. However, you could mention that you are eating to balance your brain chemistry so that you will feel less like eating while you also maintain a good mood. Once you set the discussion in that direction, no one will ask you about calories and weight. They will be more interested in how they too can eat to feel better and full.

CHAPTER FOUR

Before You Begin

By opening this book you've taken a step towards losing weight. Now you understand the major role carbohydrates play in your weight loss by controlling your appetite and your cravings. You know you need to exercise. And you probably are aware of the habits associated with overeating or eating the wrong foods that you need to change.

It's time to take a few more steps to get yourself and everyone and everything around you ready for weight loss.

Be honest. What's the real reason you want to lose weight? To look and feel sexier? Because your mother was just diagnosed with diabetes and high blood pressure? To be able to bear shopping for clothes? To be thinner than your sister-in-law? So you have more energy to play with your grandchildren? Whatever the reason, remember throughout the diet that it's important enough for you to do what it takes to achieve your weight-loss goal even though we know it won't always be easy.

Make sure the timing is right for you. Changing jobs, losing your babysitter, or gaining an unwanted relative for an extended stay may make starting a weight-loss programme just one more stressor in an already too stressful life. Losing weight is what you do for yourself, so delay starting until you have the time and mental and emotional energy required.

Before you begin, remove all temptations lurking in your house, your car, your handbag or briefcase, and your office. Favourite biscuits, crisps, salted peanuts, chocolate raisins, or whatever you can't stop eating – donate all the unopened packets to a friend and get rid of the ones she doesn't want. Don't forget to clean out the freezer; all sorts of goodies lurk behind the frozen green beans. If and when your family complains at the absence of their favourite fattening snacks, tell them that you will buy them only if they will hide them. Take the sweets off your desk at work and if possible off your colleagues' desks as well (or at least ask them to hide them). If you don't see tempting foods, you won't think of eating them.

All clothes with elastic waistbands must go. The same goes for any postmaternity clothes you're still wearing – especially if your kids are school age. The best way to tell you are losing weight is to wear clothes that feel looser as the weight comes off.

What will you wear for exercise? Make sure the fabrics breathe. This is very important if you tend to sweat. Breathable fabrics take the moisture away from your body and prevent wet T-shirt cling. Do you need to buy exercise shoes? Did you know that running shoes lose their ability to cushion your feet even if they are unused? Your feet are going to take the brunt of your exercise. Make sure that your shoes are in excellent condition and you wear socks that allow your feet to breathe, especially in warm weather.

If you haven't used your exercise equipment, like a treadmill, for a long time, you might want to have it serviced after you clean off the cobwebs. Even though exercising at home is more convenient, also check out gym facilities near your home or work. Health clubs offer a large variety of exercise options including group activities.

And now to your bathroom scales. We have clients who move their scales around the bathroom, checking for the spot that shows the lowest weight. Or they stand on the edge of the scales. Others place fingers on the wall hoping to lower the readout while some call on higher powers to reveal a low number. Leave it in one place, stand on it and track the readout.

Don't forget that you will need some support, encouragement and accountability. So tell your spouse, partner, friends, kids, relatives and colleagues that you're starting the diet. It's tough to diet alone. With others cheering you on, you'll have someone to share your success with when you reach your weight-loss goals.

Finally, decide on a reward for yourself. A weekly manicure, a weekend away, some new clothes, a massage, flowers: do whatever makes you feel good. You deserve rewards for starting, and staying on, the Good Mood Diet.

USE A PLAN THAT WORKS FOR YOU

If you want to fail at something, here's a proven way to do it: set your expectations too high. Not only will you fail to reach your goals, you'll have a built-in excuse for not succeeding.

We know that being realistic about what you want to achieve is vitally important where weight loss is concerned. That's why committing yourself to losing a certain amount of weight by a certain date – your son's graduation ceremony, for instance – can backfire. With our clients we take a much more conservative approach. That's what we did with Jan.

Eight years ago, when she was in her 30s, Jan founded and ran a successful marketing consulting business. But as her annual profits and staff size grew, so did Jan's waistline. Before she knew it she weighed 22.5 kg (3½ st) more than she ever had.

'I work 12 or 14 hours a day during the week and at least 8 hours over the weekend. That way I can get some work done without interruptions and catch up,' she told us. 'I work out once a week with a trainer, but I don't see any results. In fact, I've gained more weight recently, to the point where I am running out of clothes that fit. I'm getting desperate.'

Determined to dive into our weight-loss programme with as much gusto as she ran her business (and against our advice), Jan committed to going to the gym every day and not wavering from the diet.

Her ambitious plan to lose all the weight she'd gained in 4 months was in place for 1 day before she reverted back to her old ways. The workload never lessened and her clients and staff constantly demanded her attention. For a month, Jan's frustration grew as she recommitted to the same goals each week and never accomplished them.

Finally we convinced her to change one or two small things at a time and to follow through on them before graduating to additional changes. For the first week, her immediate goal was to go to the gym once in addition to the session with the trainer. Her second goal was to block off one 'do not disturb' hour in the day for her own focused work. That meant no calls or interruptions.

Jan tried the plan and was delighted to discover that her work did not suffer from her taking time out to go to the gym. Nor did anyone at work feel let down by her 'private' hour. Inspired by her success, she committed to another small change. The next week she added a weekly grocery-shopping trip to the workout and the blocked-off hour. That way she would have healthy foods on hand at work and at home. After 4 weeks of implementing small changes, her extra weight started to drop off at a steady rate.

Trying to change too much at once – either by carrying out too many modifications or making them too drastic – is a mistake. In most cases, big changes are unsustainable and many people soon return to their old ways. Then they feel like failures and get discouraged. Making a commitment to lose weight doesn't mean you have to drive yourself crazy. You know yourself what you can sustain. Set your own bar. That's what Molly, another client of ours, found out.

The mother of three teenagers, 47-year-old Molly worked as an administrative assistant at a local college. Over the years Molly gained weight steadily until she realized one day that nearly 18 kg (3 st) had accumulated. Understanding that she had to lose the weight and wanting to set a strong example for her 14-year-old daughter who was becoming overweight, Molly snapped into action.

Her initial success was remarkable. She followed the eating plan religiously and went to her women-only gym five times a week before work. That workout was supplemented with 15 minutes on an elliptical trainer at work and doing extra exercises with hand weights. Her new, disciplined habits paid off with a 2.75-kg (6-lb) weight loss in 3 weeks.

Yet despite her joy over her accomplishment, Molly was exhausted from waking up earlier every day and still juggling the demands of family and work. Then she was appointed co-chair of an annual fundraising event, which put even more demands on her time.

To help her cope, we suggested that she be vigilant about scheduling her time so that meal planning and at least three weekly exercise sessions did not get dropped.

But the next week Molly was discouraged. She had gained a pound and told us that she hadn't made time for weekly food shopping. Meals at home weren't well planned and she felt so rushed that she neglected to carry proper snacks and meals with her on days when she knew she'd have no other way of staying on the eating plan. She had made it to the gym only once. Subsequent weeks were worse. One week she did not go to the gym at all because her kids were behind with their homework. Additionally, they had overscheduled their social activities, thereby requiring Molly to drive them around to various places. Consequently she was too tired to exercise in the morning.

As a result, she reverted back to eating whatever was at hand when she was hungry, including the cakes her colleagues brought in several times a week. After gaining back nearly all the weight she'd lost, Molly was angry with herself for deviating from her initially perfect execution. But given her demanding family and work responsibilities, Molly's all-or-nothing approach was clearly unsustainable.

When she finally realized that her method wasn't working, Molly sat down and wrote out the regular schedule of each family member. Then she reviewed it with her family. She included time for her own exercise, food shopping and meal planning. She also filled out a timeline with the co-chair of the fundraising event so she could pace herself and not become overwhelmed with extra work pressure. Molly restarted the diet in a sustainable way, and this time it worked.

Remember the tortoise and the hare? Small, steady steps work for weight loss, too.

FOCUS ON THE PROCESS, NOT THE RESULT

Many of our clients want to lose significant amounts of weight. As we support their goals, we also advise them to concentrate on what they are doing day by day, and not on the final result.

Losing weight takes time and everyone's body is different. While clients usually shed between 0.5 and 1 kg (1–2 lb) a week, some people lose more, some less. Sometimes more is lost initially and then the loss levels off a little. For many people this can be frustrating; they think they won't be able to reach their goal. That is not the case. Just as every day in your life is different, so is weight loss.

You can't control how quickly you will reach your goal, but you can control how you carry out your plan. If you follow what you are supposed to do, you will lose weight and reach your goal.

Achieving a big goal is the culmination of completing a series of small, doable bits. Focusing on what you will do in 1 day or 1 week, for example, as opposed to what you will accomplish in 6 months time, is a lot more manageable mentally.

A number of techniques will help you to focus. Constant reminders will reinforce what you are doing and keep you from straying. Here's what some of our clients did.

Alan weighed himself every morning as a reminder that he was on a diet. He knew that his weight could fluctuate from day to day. 'As an engineer, I know the value of recording a trend. I don't get emotional about the numbers on the scales as long as the overall trend is down. I use it as a tool to help me stay on track,' he explained.

Patty, an estate agent, set a timer on her mobile phone to remind her of when it was time for snacks and meals. Otherwise she would get caught up in business with clients all day and forget to eat until she was famished. 'When I'm running on empty, I know I'll fill up on whatever I can grab. I rely on my mobile phone for practically everything else – why shouldn't it remind me of when to eat?' she pointed out.

Every Tuesday and Friday Louise met a friend for an early morning power yoga class. Eventually they befriended the teacher and the other students, who applauded their weight loss. 'The support we receive is positively addictive,' Louise said.

Tom, a busy doctor, asked his receptionist to order him the same lunch every day (a large mixed green salad with grilled chicken, no dressing). That way he was not tempted to look at the menu and order something more fattening. 'I like not having to deal with temptation when I am eating. Having my meal planned ahead of time makes lunch much easier,' he told us.

Pamela and her friend Bethany, who live across the country from each other, exchanged daily e-mail reports on their eating and exercise. Their messages also maintained an open channel of communication through which to vent stresses and share successes in other areas of their lives. Doing so kept them on track. 'Just knowing that I would have to tell Bethany that I ate some biscuits makes me think twice before eating them,' Pamela confessed.

After claiming that he was watching his eating, Walter discovered that keeping a food journal was the only way to really stay on target. 'At first it made me realize I overeat at dinnertime. Now it makes me more mindful at every meal and I keep an eye on portion sizes,' he stated.

Emily and her husband, recently married and both overweight, ate dinner out often. When they both started our diet, they made a visit to the local farmers' market, as well as a supermarket, a weekly habit. They enjoyed planning their meals and bringing leftovers to work, which saved money. Then they started a new tradition of dinner parties in their home. Their friends didn't even realize that they too were eating according to the Good Mood Diet.

David also ate out frequently and made up his mind to stick to the Good Mood Diet wherever he was eating lunch or dinner. 'The interesting thing is that I never feel out of place or ill at ease,' he told us. 'The truth is that making a stand for what I want to do for myself makes me feel really good.'

Focus on making small, consistent changes to build a track record of success. Add one or two things at a time. If you like, you can drop one before adding another. Stick with each change for at least a week (preferably 2) to give it a chance to work.

HABIT FORMING

You didn't become overweight overnight. It took time to put on the extra weight and it also took time for you to develop the habits that put it on. Some of these habits may, to some extent, define who you are. You may not want to lose them because they've become comfortable and familiar. It is especially hard to replace these overeating habits when eating is comforting and even entertaining.

For instance, opening a bag of crisps or ordering a pizza in the face of stress could be something you do without even thinking about it. Or you may just assume that you will overeat in social situations like get-togethers with family or friends or dinners with clients.

But changing one habit doesn't mean giving up all sources of comfort when you are upset. The Good Mood Diet programme focuses on specific foods that really do comfort you for hours. And giving up eating and drinking too many calories does not mean that you will no longer have a social life. Instead, it means learning how to eat and drink so you can lose weight and keep it off.

For instance, eating a serotonin-friendly snack before happy hour will greatly reduce the likelihood that you'll want to indulge in bar food or more than one drink. Ordering a nonalcoholic beverage, or limiting yourself to one wine spritzer and then switching to a nonalcoholic, low-calorie beverage, will allow you to socialize and not feel left out. And if you've been invited for a meal at someone else's house, offer to bring a side dish, a main course or fruit or other fat-free item for dessert. You'll stay on the diet and still be able to enjoy the meal with your dining companions.

Changing habits takes time, sometimes more time than you expect. If practised daily, a new habit takes 2 or more weeks to become a regular part of your life. It can take longer if the new habit is used less frequently. Sometimes establishing new habits requires that you make renewed commitments to the change. We have found with our clients that it can take up to 6 to 8 weeks for a new habit to become second nature. However, when a new habit is clearly associated with a positive result like weight loss, it's easily, and more quickly, adopted.

But, in the face of difficulty, most people will revert back to the comfort of their old habits. Those usually include not ensuring that proper food is available for meals and snacks, skipping exercise sessions, and eating whatever is in sight.

Establishing new habits is challenging, so it's important to remember that committing to making a change means making a commitment to yourself. You must do whatever it takes to honour that pledge, at least as much as – or even more than – it takes to honour promises made to others. There is nothing wrong with putting yourself first. (Don't think that's right? Well, airlines do. Their safety instructions direct you to put on your own oxygen mask first and then help others.)

So remind yourself of the new habits you are establishing and keep repeating them. Soon you will have control over your actions no matter what else is going on.

If weight loss is important to you, it must be a priority in your mind, on your calendar, and in your actions. Everything that you decide to do to lose weight may require changing how you think about using your time. And it may require changing your lifestyle.

FREQUENTLY ASKED QUESTIONS

When is the best time to start a diet?

Many people find the winter a hard time to diet because the lack of sunlight can depress mood and increase appetite, and it can also be hard to exercise if the weather is bad. The Good Mood Diet works in every season because it increases serotonin, the body's natural mood energizer. It will keep your appetite and mood under control – and that means you will be more likely to be motivated to exercise, whether you do it indoors or outdoors.

My husband and I like to travel and he plans the trips around restaurants he would like to try. We tend to go out for a large lunch and a larger dinner and I always return over 3 kg [½ st] heavier. Should I wait until I come back to start the diet? Or should I begin it before we leave, lose the weight and then accept the fact that I will gain it back again?

Start your diet before your trip and make sure that you establish an exercise routine along with your eating plan. If your body is accustomed to exercising several times a week you will want to continue to work out, even while you're on your trip. Then do this: speak to your husband about your concerns regarding gaining back the weight you are working so hard to lose. See if you can compromise on how you spend your holiday. For instance, walk for a couple of hours between meals or use the hotel's health club. If you visit cities where walking is part of seeing and enjoying the excitement of the place (like London or Paris), then you will be able to burn off the extra calories from lavish meals.

Restaurants need not be a prescription for diet disaster, either. Although you may not be able to follow the structure of the diet programme, you can order wisely and avoid foods that are very high in fat. Moreover, you do not have to eat everything on your plate. Your husband may be happy to help himself to some of your selection. That way he will be able to sample more from the menu. If you order appetizers for lunch rather than the main course, the calories you ingest will be lower as well.

*My friends and I go away for a long weekend every summer to the
holiday home of one friend's grandparents. We eat and drink and
just take it easy. I had planned to wait until after that to start the
diet, but spring is a good time for me to lose weight, so I would
prefer to start the diet before my trip. But how do I handle all the
eating and drinking we will be doing on the trip without gaining
weight and without spoiling the fun?*

As you are going with friends, enlist their support for your weight-
loss efforts. Tell them ahead of time that you are following a
structured food plan that does not permit more than a minimal
amount of alcohol and requires healthy meals on a consistent
schedule. Insist that your eating plans should not interfere with what
they do and that anyway, you are coming to see them, not the food
and alcohol that will be on hand.

Take food with you or go to the supermarket when you arrive and
make sure you buy the foods you should be eating, including snacks
along with the pasta or potatoes or rice to cook for dinner. If you go
out to eat, you can still follow the diet plan (see page 115 for
restaurant guidelines).

You may be surprised by how much your friends help you with
your diet. After all, they are your friends.

*I am in sales and taking clients to dinner several times a week is an
integral part of my job. How can I hold back from eating and
drinking along with everyone else? Won't it adversely affect my
business relationship with them?*

Is it bad business to eat in a healthy manner? Are you being less
than effective as a salesperson if you are frugal in your alcohol
consumption so you can be in charge and control the conversation
and communicate information? Your mandate is to entertain your
clients and you can do this, as a gracious host, without eating and
drinking as they do. Order drinks and wines as before; you do not
have to consume them. If you feel you must order a mixed drink,
just sip it. When the wine comes, do the same thing. Remember
that your primary task is to carry out business, which is why your
meal is on an expense account. Only restaurant critics are paid
to eat.

I have a bad knee and cannot exercise without pain. My doctor says I
need a knee replacement but I must lose weight first. You say I should
plan on exercising to lose weight. So should I still go on the diet?

Yes. You will drop weight faster if you can exercise, but reducing
your calorie intake and controlling your appetite with the Good
Mood Diet will allow you to lose weight easily and consistently. As
you lose weight, you will find that your ability to walk will improve
because there will be less pressure on your knee. Ask your doctor or
physiotherapist if you can walk with a cane, swim or perform some
non-weight-bearing exercises.

I'm a schoolteacher, and I thought I would wait until school was out
before starting the diet and remain on it until school begins again
in the autumn. But I always gain weight during the school year, so I
always feel hopeless about losing weight.

Many teachers have used the Good Mood Diet, and they have been
able to lose weight during both the school year and holidays. You
will find that the carbohydrate snacks are effective in curbing your
appetite before lunch and renewing your stamina in the afternoon.

I work as an assistant to a tax accountant. Every year around the tax
deadline our office gets crazy and in the past I have gained a lot of
weight at this time. Should I start the diet late in January so I can lose
some weight before gaining it again during the busy period?

It is a good idea to start the diet before all your time is consumed by
work. If you give yourself 5 or 6 weeks to become familiar with the
meal and snack plans and develop an exercise plan prior to your
busy period, then you will lose weight and increase your stamina.

However, once you start to almost live in the office, it will be more
difficult to follow the diet and to get in enough exercise. The answer is
to plan ahead. Choose foods that you can take into the office for quick
meals. For instance, canned tuna or salmon; fruit; cut raw vegetables;
low-fat or fat-free cottage cheese or yogurt; and microwaveable rice are
convenient. Also bring diet-plan snacks to work; they will prevent you
from chewing your exhaustion away on high-calorie foods.

You may not lose any more weight until the last tax return is
finished, but you will prevent yourself from gaining any weight.

PART TWO

THE PROGRAMME

Snack Your Way to Serotonin Power

Most diet plans start with a meal plan. The Good Mood Diet programme starts with a snack plan because snacks are the most important component of the diet. The type of snacks and when you should snack are designed to increase the serotonin in your brain as quickly as possible and to maintain this level throughout the diet. You will use serotonin power, not willpower, to control your eating.

YOU MUST SNACK

During the first two weeks of the diet, the Serotonin Surge phase, you will eat three carbohydrate snacks a day. The resulting increase in serotonin will decrease your appetite and stop overeating.

In weeks 3 through 8, the Serotonin Balance phase, you will eat two snacks a day to maintain your more balanced serotonin levels.

By week 9 and beyond, the Serotonin Control phase, you will be able to control your appetite by eating one snack a day.

Your snacks will always be carbohydrate but the amount will change as you move through the phases of the diet.

Phase 1: Serotonin Surge Snacking Schedule

Snack 1: Eat an hour before lunch.

Snack 2: Eat mid- to late afternoon, 3 or 4 hours after lunch.

Snack 3: Eat in mid-evening, 2 or 3 hours after dinner.

Phase 1 snacks, for both men and women, should contain:

Carbohydrate: 30 to 40 grams of sweet, starchy, or a combination of sweet and starchy carbohydrates – unless you have 6.8 kg (15 lb) or less to lose. In that case, make sure your snack does not have any more than 30 grams of carbohydrate.

Fat: No more than 1 to 3 grams (avoid trans fat)

Protein: No more than 5 grams, preferably less

Calories: No more than 180

Good snacks for phase 1 are low-fat or fat-free breakfast cereals or crackers. See page 66 for a list of snack suggestions.

Phase 2: Serotonin Balance Snacking Schedule

Snack 1: Eat an hour before lunch.

Snack 2: Eat mid- to late afternoon, 3 or 4 hours after lunch.

Phase 2 snacks should be the same as phase 1 snacks.

Phase 3: Serotonin Control Snacking Schedule

Snack 1: Eat mid- to late afternoon, 3 or 4 hours after lunch.

Phase 3 snacks, for both men and women, should contain:

Carbohydrate: 20 to 25 grams of sweet, starchy, or a combination of sweet and starchy carbohydrates

Fat: No more than 1 to 2 grams (avoid trans fat)

Protein: No more than 3 grams, preferably less

Calories: 100 to 120

See page 67 for snack suggestions.

HOW TO EAT THE SNACKS

Consume your snacks within 10 minutes after starting to eat them. Munching on them over a longer time will result in slower serotonin production. Expect the appetite-suppressing, mood-enhancing effects to take place in approximately 30 minutes during the first 3 to 4 weeks of the diet and then in 20 minutes thereafter.

Eat the snacks on an empty stomach or at least 3 hours after eating a meal that contains protein. If you eat the snack while your stomach is still digesting protein, the protein will interfere with serotonin production.

Prevent yourself from overeating by using prepackaged foods. If you need to pack your own snack, like breakfast cereal or rice cakes, put it in a ziploc bag and then put the bag in your briefcase or in a special place in the kitchen hours before you'll want it. An open box or bag is an invitation to eat too much.

The snacks will increase serotonin more quickly when you have lost 4.5 kg (10 lb) or more. This is because as you lose weight, you gain insulin sensitivity. Insulin will work faster to get tryptophan into your brain and make new serotonin.

CHOOSE THE CORRECT SNACK

The first step in choosing a snack for any phase of the diet programme is to read the nutrition facts label. That will tell you how much carbohydrate and how many calories are in a serving and how much added fat and protein you will be getting. Here is a (somewhat abbreviated) sample label.

If you picked Snack-a-Jack Chocolate and Orange rice cakes for your snack, you would eat 3 rice cakes for your Surge and Balance phase snacks and 2 rice cakes for your Control snack.

Sometimes a snack choice will not meet our guidelines perfectly. That is all right. The snack can be a little over or under in carbohydrate and calorie content and still work to increase serotonin and help you lose weight.

Nutrition Information

Chocolate & orange flavour rice & corn snacks

	Per 15 g cake:
Energy	250 kJ/59 kcal
Protein	0.8 g
Carbohydrate	12.5 g
Fat	0.7 g

There is one thing you must keep in mind when choosing your snacks. They are not a treat. They are a treatment to increase your serotonin level. If there were some way of getting more serotonin into your brain with a pill, we would recommend it. But there isn't. You must rely on the only option nature gives you, and that is carbohydrates. You need just enough to take the edge off your appetite. Too many calories will sabotage your weight-loss efforts, particularly during the first two phases of the diet plan. Choose snacks that do not tempt you – the more boring, the better.

For example, if the choice is between plain shredded wheat squares and oat clusters that contain bits of nuts, raisins and sweetened oat flakes, opt for the shredded wheat squares. As long as the foods have nutrition labels, you will be able to make wise choices. Here are a few examples of snacks that we consider to be resistible (that is, not tempting):

Bread sticks

Breakfast cereals

Dutch crispbakes

English muffin, wholewheat

Finn Crisp crackers

Hot chocolate, fat-free

Matzo crackers, white or wholewheat

Pitta bread, small

Raisin bread

Reduced-fat table water biscuits

Rice cakes, plain

Saltine crackers

When you know that you can control the size of the snacks you are eating, you can increase their variety and palatability. Always check labels but here are a few possibilities:

Cereal bars, low-fat

Marshmallows

Popcorn, air-popped

Japanese rice crackers

Rice cakes, sweetened/flavoured

Turkish delight (not chocolate covered)

Tip: Do you live near a good bakery? Buy a small roll of chewy multigrain bread for a snack. You will be surprised by how delicious a piece of fresh bread can taste without a spread.

When you reach Serotonin Control, the final phase of the Good Mood Diet, your cravings will be in check and you'll be able to enjoy a greater variety of snacks without overeating them – even if some of them may have tempted you before. Just be sure to pay close attention to phase 3 portion sizes. The snacks have fewer calories (no more than 120) and less carbohydrate than those allowed in the earlier parts of the diet. Here are a few possibilities.

Sorbet, low-fat frozen yogurt or Skinny Cow low- or no-fat frozen desserts

Low-fat packaged cakes, such as less-than-3%-fat carrot cake slices and lower calorie biscuits such as fig rolls, garibaldi and light rich tea

Low-calorie fruit and muesli bars (avoid those with nuts as these will be too high in fat)

Liquorice, sugar-free fruit chews and other fat-free sweets (don't forget to keep track of the calories – no fat does not mean no calories)

100-calorie packs of crackers (or make up your own for work)

Strawberries dipped in Marshmallow Fluff (a marshmallow spread) and a few chocolate chips

Be sure to read nutrition labels for calorie, protein, carbohydrate and fat content. Some of our clients tell us that these once-in-a-while treats keep them on the Good Mood Diet and ultimately help them reach their weight-loss goals. But do not indulge in these treats unless you know you can restrict yourself to the proper serving sizes!

HEARING THE SNACK ALARM

You may not always be able to snack on time. On some days, lunchtime will come around before you remember or have the time to eat your late-morning snack. If this happens, have your snack and wait 30 minutes before eating your lunch. If it's really late and beyond your normal mealtime, skip your snack and just eat your lunch.

You will notice, especially at the beginning of the diet programme, that it is much harder to stick to the diet portions when you do not have your appetite-suppressing snack ahead of time. Almost all of our clients have forgotten or were unable to snack at the correct time at least once while on the programme, and they all told us the same thing. All related a variation of 'I ate enough food to make me full, but I wasn't satisfied and kept looking for something sweet or crunchy to eat after the meal was over.'

To avoid missing your snack time, keep a snack schedule handy. Stick it on your calendar, computer, refrigerator, car dashboard or mobile phone.

As the diet proceeds, you will become more and more sensitive to your brain's signals. There may be times during the diet, as well as during the post-diet phase, when your need for serotonin, and therefore for snacks, increases.

For instance, during the dark days of autumn and winter, your carbohydrate cravings and need for serotonin may increase due to the lack of sunlight. Or if your medication is changed or you experience a particularly bad bout of PMS, you may find yourself with a more intense craving for carbohydrates. If this happens, increase the number of snacks to up to three a day, until you feel that your cravings and your mood are under control once more.

As you lose weight, your cravings will become less noticeable or may disappear altogether. This indicates that your brain finally contains sufficient serotonin to turn off your appetite and stabilize your mood. By the time you reach the Control phase of the diet programme, you may find yourself not needing to snack every single day. You can skip your snack for a day or two, but be vigilant in listening to your brain's signals that you need serotonin. They include difficulty in controlling your eating, not feeling full after a meal, craving carbohydrates, and increased moodiness or impatience. If this happens, go back to the Control snack schedule you were on.

GIVE YOUR BRAIN AN EXTRA BOOST

Even though the carbohydrate snack will help your brain make you feel calm and relaxed, you can also consciously assist in the process. During the interval in which the brain begins to make new serotonin, immediately after you eat a snack, focus your mind on a pleasurable activity to enhance the serotonin effect.

Do

Read a chapter of a fast-paced book you keep nearby.

Make a phone call to a friend.

Surf the Web for sites that appeal to you.

Listen to some music (with earphones if necessary).

Send an e-mail to a friend or family member.

Read a magazine article.

Go outside for 5 to 10 minutes.

Window-shop or try on shoes.

Listen to a chapter from a book on tape.

Knit a few rows on a project in progress.

Meditate for 2 minutes.

Do some gentle stretching.

Drink a glass of water or a cup of unsweetened herbal tea.

Look at photos on your computer or in an album.

Brush the dog or cat.

Feed your goldfish.

Pick a few flowers, or a few weeds, from your garden.

Thumb through a catalogue (anything but food).

Look through your tie collection.

Don't

Go to the supermarket.

Lie on the sofa and watch cookery programmes.

Leaf through cookbooks or cooking magazines.

Sit in the kitchen.

Feed your kids a snack (set it out earlier, if need be).

Start making supper. Cooking will simply make it easier to eat.

Weigh yourself.

WHEN SNACKING WON'T STOP

Sometimes stress, too many teenagers to cope with or too much work erodes your control over your eating and impulse trumps patience. Even though you know that your appetite will be subdued 20 or so minutes after you finish your snack, you can't stop eating.

An intensely sweet snack not only causes a quick and powerful surge of serotonin, it is also virtually impossible to overeat. You can snack on so-called energy gels called GO gel or High 5, which were originally developed for endurance athletes. You can find these foods in sporting goods and health-food shops and online. Check labels and aim to consume between 100 and 200 calories of these foods.

SNACKING BEYOND THE DIET

After you complete the diet and your weight is stable, you should continue to snack in the afternoon. Although you may not feel the need to snack on some days, most of the time you will find yourself feeling a slight increase in your appetite and decrease in your good mood late in the afternoon. This seems to be the universal carbohydrate-craving time. For reasons we do not yet understand, there seems to be a need for your brain – and the brains of millions of other people – to make serotonin at this time of day.

Years ago, researchers noticed that there seemed to be a change in mental and emotional energy late in the afternoon.[1-2] Regardless of their weight, clients reported feeling some of the behavioural changes listed below.

- Moodiness
- Difficulty in concentrating
- Feeling tired
- Impatience

- Feeling restless and/or bored, yet not sure what to do
- Grumpiness
- Feeling overwhelmed
- Feeling a need to relax, unwind and de-stress
- Feeling an intense desire to eat something sweet or starchy

These behavioural changes pointed to the brain needing more serotonin late in the afternoon. When this need for serotonin was satisfied by eating a small carbohydrate snack, people felt their mental alertness and emotional well-being were restored.

This need for afternoon serotonin will remain even after the diet is over. That's why it is so important to keep snacking in the afternoon.

THE POWER OF SNACKS TO BOOST WILLPOWER

Richard, a business executive whose constant travel and perpetual stress had added around 36 kg (over 5 st) to his rather short frame, was sure that he would never lose weight if he ate snacks. He told us that snacking was the cause of his weight problem.

'I have no control over my snacking,' he stated. 'Willpower means nothing to me. I know that if I snack, I will overdo it.'

Still, he was willing to give the diet a try, and he alternated between eating the diet-plan snacks when he was at home and drinking Serotrim, a portion-controlled carbohydrate beverage formulated especially for our diet plan, when he was travelling.

After 3 weeks and a 4-kg (9-lb) weight loss, he reported that he had to remind himself to eat lunch because the late-morning snack was so effective in eliminating thoughts about food. Snacking reduced his appetite so effectively that he wanted to skip his afternoon snack so he could overeat at a famous restaurant he was going to that evening. We told him to eat his afternoon snack so he would not be vulnerable to doing more than just sampling the restaurant foods and suggested that he take home whatever foods he was not hungry enough to eat at dinner. He followed our advice and enjoyed the meal immensely, especially because he did not overeat.

Richard's successful weight loss showed that eating the correct snacks at the appropriate times can indeed support weak willpower.

To adapt a well-known expression, a snack a day will keep the grumpiness away (as well as the weight).

Ellen, a client who worked at a high-pressure accountancy firm, is typical of someone who experienced the need for an afternoon snack before, during and after her diet.

'I spend most of the day poring over tax codes and income-tax forms and I enjoy doing this work,' she said. 'But every day around 4 o'clock my functioning comes to a halt. The numbers run into each other and I read the same paragraph a dozen times without understanding it. Before I started on the diet, I used to go into the office kitchen and help myself to a few handfuls of cookies. I found that in about 30 minutes my head would clear, the restlessness would disappear, and I could work for several more hours. Of course my shape disappeared as well. I went up two dress sizes since starting at this firm.'

After Ellen went on the Good Mood Diet, she was able to get back into her original dress size in a few months. Then she assumed that she would stop snacking since she no longer had to lose weight. But we explained to her that her brain hadn't changed and she would continue to experience the late-afternoon dip in serotonin. By then she knew how to snack in a calorie- and portion-controlled way. When she was assured that she was not in danger of regaining weight by continuing her afternoon snack time, Ellen was relieved.

'I really need the snack, and now I realize that eating it is something my brain is telling me to do. And I'm glad to listen to my brain,' she said.

FREQUENTLY ASKED QUESTIONS

Won't I gain weight if I snack on sugary snacks?

You won't as long as the snacks are fat-free or very low in fat. If you pay attention to portion size, the snacks will help you lose weight. Just remember to brush your teeth, chew sugarless gum or rinse with mouthwash afterward.

How can you suggest snacks like sweet breakfast cereals rather than wholegrain cereals? Shouldn't we always eat whole grains and limit our sugar consumption?

Whole grain snack and meal foods are the most nutritious, and you can always choose them over refined options. But snack portions are small and their purpose is to elevate serotonin levels in the brain, not to act as a source of nutrition for the body. Although your brain gets a boost of serotonin after eating unrefined carbohydrates, refined, starchy carbohydrates and sugar also raise serotonin levels effectively, which is why we allow them on the diet. Also, many dieters feel deprived without sweet foods – to the point where they would abort their weight-loss efforts if they couldn't have them. However, do nourish your body with the nutrients in whole grains by choosing them for meals and snacks as often as possible, especially when you do not crave sugary foods.

You say that I won't overeat snacks on this diet – but I have been known to binge on bran cereal. I do not trust myself to eat any snack, no matter how bland or uninteresting. How can I control myself?

Once you allow yourself to eat the correct amount of carbohydrate and then wait until the serotonin is made, you will feel more confident that the snacks will control your appetite. However, if you do not trust yourself to start this process using real foods, you can try the energy gels described on page 70 for a week. Because these foods are designed to be digested faster than food, you will feel the effect sooner. In our experience, no one ever binges on them.

Can't I drink sugary fruit drinks for a snack?

Sugary beverages do not work as snacks. Most contain corn syrup solids that are mostly fructose, which is fruit sugar. Fructose does not cause significant amounts of insulin to be released, so no serotonin will be produced.

The glycaemic index, or GI seems to be really popular. Don't I have to stay away from foods that have a high GI?

The glycaemic index measures how quickly glucose levels rise in the blood after eating. A number of our clients voiced concerns about these blood sugar spikes.

However, unless someone is diabetic, the carbohydrate amounts in our snacks will not cause significant blood sugar swings. Insulin in the absence of diabetes is extremely effective at maintaining blood glucose levels within the normal range.

The Good Mood Diet

This unique diet will allow the power of your brain chemistry to control your cravings. The simple-to-follow plan, chock-full of delicious, comforting foods, will control your appetite and balance your mood while you lose weight.

PHASE 1: SEROTONIN SURGE

It is particularly important for dieters who have either avoided or minimized their carbohydrate intake to stay on this first phase for the entire 2 weeks. The same is true of dieters who are on antidepressants. The goal is to make you aware that your brain, and not your stomach, can shut off your eating.

YOUR SEROTONIN SURGE MEALS AND SNACKS

- Breakfast: Protein, carbohydrate and fruit or fruit juice. If you prefer, the fruit or fruit juice can be eaten at some other time of the day.
- Snack: 1 hour before lunch
- Lunch: Protein and vegetables
- Snack: 3 or 4 hours after lunch
- Dinner: Carbohydrate and vegetables
- Snack: 2 or 3 hours after dinner

Serotonin Surge Breakfast Guidelines

Breakfast stays the same throughout all phases of the diet. It consists of one serving of protein, a starchy carbohydrate and fruit. The sample breakfast menus in the three diet phases are interchangeable.

If you are in the habit of adding cream and sugar to your coffee or tea and you can accept these alternatives, switch to skimmed milk and artificial sweetener. If you must have cream and sugar, add no more than 1 teaspoon of cream or 1 coffee-shop-size container and 1 packet of sugar to each cup.

Non-traditional breakfast foods such as chicken, beef and tuna are also options (if you have some meat left over from the previous night's dinner it is a very convenient option – and is surprisingly tasty with toast). Keep portion sizes to about 30 g (1 oz) for women and 45–60 g (1½–2 oz) for men.

Protein	Women (serving size)	Men (serving size)
Cottage cheese, low-fat (chive, pineapple, plain)	115 g (4 oz)	170 g (6 oz)
Egg, any style (use nonstick spray for frying or scrambling)	1 large egg	2 large eggs
Ham, very lean (50 calories/slice)	2 slices	3 slices
Milk, skimmed (lactose-free milk or soya milk are good options for people with lactose intolerance)	240 ml (8 fl oz)	300 ml (10 fl oz)
Ricotta, fat-free or low-fat	125 g (4½ oz)	185 g (6½ oz)
Smoked salmon	2 slices	3 slices
Vegetarian sausages or burgers (at least 10 grams protein each)	1	2
Yogurt, flavoured or natural, fat-free or low-fat	240 g (8 oz)	360 g (12½ oz)

Ignore the carbohydrate listed on nutrition labels for some dairy products, such as yogurt. It doesn't count as a carbohydrate serving. Choose wholegrain carbohydrates if possible. Cereal eaten at breakfast should be made of whole grains, high in fibre if possible, and low in fat and sugar. Reserve the sugary low-fat or fat-free cereals for snacks.

Carbohydrate	Women (serving size)	Men (serving size)
Bread	1 regular or 2 diet slices	2 regular or 4 diet slices
Cereals, cold, low-fat	30 g (1 oz)	40 g (1⅓ oz)
Crackers, wholegrain	4	6
English muffin, wholegrain	1 regular	1 large
Hot cereal	30 g (1 oz)	40 g (1¼ oz)
Pitta bread, wholemeal	1 small	1 regular

Eat one fruit a day. The amounts given below equal one serving for both men and women.

Fruit	Women/Men (serving size)
Apple	1 medium
Banana	½ medium
Berries	145 g (5 oz)
Citrus juice	150 ml (5 fl oz)
Dried fruit	75 g (2½ oz)
Grapefruit	½ fruit
Kiwi	2 small
Melon	⅛ fruit
Orange	1 medium
Pear	1 medium
Pineapple	125 g (4½ oz)
Tangerine/satsuma	2 small

Seratonin Surge Lunch Guidelines

Lunch is the main protein meal of the day. During the Serotonin Surge phase, women should eat 115 g (4 oz) and men should eat 170 g (6 oz) of protein. Note: some sources of protein (e.g. cottage cheese) are less dense or 'complete' than fish or meat, so the serving size is higher.

Protein	Women (serving size)	Men (serving size)
Fish/meat/pork/poultry/seafood	115 g (4 oz)	170 g (6 oz)
Cottage cheese, low-fat	230 g (8 oz)	340 g (12 oz)
Deli meat, very low fat	3 slices	5 slices
Egg-white omelette	5 or 6 egg whites	7 or 8 egg whites
Tuna or salmon, canned in water*	185-g can	185-g can
Tofu, firm silken-style	180 g (6½ oz)	275 g (9¼ oz)
Vegetarian burgers (look for at least 15 grams protein/burger)	2	3

*Each can contains about 115 g (4 oz) of fish; the rest is water. Men should add additional fish to make up the difference.

Vegetables	Women/Men (serving size)
Any combination of vegetables	150–200 g (5½–7 oz) or more
Carrots or beetroots*	Limit to 200 g (7 oz)**

*These vegetables are restricted because they are dense.

**More than this will provide too many calories.

Serotonin Surge Dinner Guidelines

The Serotonin Surge dinner is a complex carbohydrate and vegetable meal with whatever low-fat or fat-free ingredients you wish to add during preparation. The servings may seem too large for a diet, but remember that the carbohydrate is the main dish. The portions are calculated to make sure you feel satisfied.

If you want to taste a protein dish served to others, take only a bite. More may interfere with serotonin production. However, beef, chicken, or fish stock or soup can be used as the cooking or flavour base of your food. Their protein content is too small to affect serotonin synthesis.

Do not hesitate to mix carbohydrates together. For instance, you can add peas, corn or beans to a rice dish. Many of the recipes in this book combine two or more of these carbohydrates. If the dish also contains vegetables, measure the vegetables separately so you serve yourself the correct amount of carbohydrate.

Carbohydrate	Women (serving size)	Men (serving size)
Basic grains and pulses, cooked: barley, bulgur wheat, chickpeas and other beans, couscous, buckwheat, lentils, millet, pasta, polenta, quinoa, rice, split peas	230 g (8 oz)	300 g (10½ oz)
Bread (30 g/1 oz slice)	4 slices	6 slices
Corn tortilla (15 cm/6 in)*	4	6
Flour tortilla (25 cm/10 in)	1½	2
Pitta, wholemeal or white 60 g (2 oz)	2	3
Potato, sweet or white (raw weight)	340 g (12 oz)	455 g (1 lb)
Sweetcorn**	300 g (10½ oz)	455 g (1 lb)

*Corn tortillas are low in calories. Use them as wraps and fill with rice and beans or other carbohydrate combinations.

**Sweetcorn makes a good dinner carb when combined with other starches like rice or couscous or when used as filling in a wrap.

Vegetables	Women/Men (serving size)
Any combination of vegetables	150–200 g (5½–7 oz) or more
Carrots or beetroots*	Limit to 200 g (7 oz)**

*These vegetables are restricted because they are dense.

**More than this will provide too many calories.

For both men and women, 150–200 g (5½–7 oz) of vegetables as listed above should be eaten at dinner. This can be a single vegetable or a mixture of vegetables and either raw or cooked. Make selections from among the great variety of vegetables to keep your meals interesting and to get a broad range of nutrients.

Serotonin Surge Phase Recap

The amount of protein consumed at lunch is highest during the first phase of the Good Mood Diet because no protein is included in dinner. Lunch provides you with most of the protein that you must eat every day. Don't skimp on it.

If you can't or won't eat vegetables at lunch, have a serving of fruit instead.

Dinner consists of complex carbohydrates (pasta, rice, beans or polenta) and vegetables.

If you do not feel like eating anything after dinner, skip the third snack. A calorie not eaten is a calorie not eaten.

Sample Menus for the Serotonin Surge Phase

Recipes for the menu suggestions offered for each phase of the Good Mood Diet can be found in Chapter 14. Recipes are noted with an asterisk (*). For serving sizes, see the guidelines on pages 75 to 78. Also check out Chapter 12, which is full of suggestions for delicious, easy meals in minutes.

Day 1 Serotonin Surge

Breakfast

Low-fat cottage cheese

Wholegrain English muffin with 1 teaspoon all-fruit jam

Banana, blueberries or strawberries

Snack, 1 hour before lunch

40 g/1¼ oz wholegrain Cheerios

Lunch

Chef's Salad (lettuce, tomatoes, turkey, ham, boiled egg, a little cheese)

Snack, 3 hours after lunch

1 bag caramel Snack-a-Jack minis

Dinner

Baked potato with topping of choice

Lemon Garlic Spinach*

Cucumber, red and green pepper, and cherry tomato salad with choice of dressing*

Snack, 2 hours after dinner

1 cup low-fat instant hot chocolate with 2 marshmallows

Day 2 Serotonin Surge

Breakfast

½ grapefruit

Rye bread

Smoked salmon

Snack, 1 hour before lunch

5 small Japanese rice crackers

Lunch

Sautéed Scallops*

Steamed fresh or frozen broccoli or green beans

Snack, 3 hours after lunch

2 Finn Crisp crackers

1 teaspoon Marshmallow Fluff or jelly (optional)

Dinner

Pad Thai Salad*

Steamed mixed vegetables

Snack, 2 hours after dinner

45 g (1½ oz) Kashi Honey 7-grain Cereal

Day 3 Serotonin Surge

Breakfast

Orange or grapefruit juice

Scrambled eggs or omelette cooked with 1 wedge Laughing Cow low-fat cheese

Thinly sliced wholemeal toast and 1 teaspoon all-fruit jam

Snack, 1 hour before lunch

45 g (1½ oz) Oatibix Bitesize Cereal (sultana and apple)

Lunch

Cheeseburger*

Coleslaw*

Snack, 3 hours after lunch

1–2 low-fat cereal bars

Dinner

Spaghetti with Roasted Courgette and Onion*

Tossed green salad with Italian Dressing*

Snack, 2 hours after dinner

1 bag caramel Snack-a-Jack minis

PHASE 2: SEROTONIN BALANCE

The meals and snacks in this part of the diet programme will maintain the high serotonin levels that were produced by the Serotonin Surge phase. By the time you start this part of the diet programme, the effects of a low-carbohydrate diet, antidepressant use or emotional stress on serotonin levels should be remedied. For this reason, the evening snack is eliminated and a small amount of protein is added to the evening meal.

If at any time during this middle phase of the diet you feel an increase in your need for carbohydrate to control your appetite or reduce your stress, go back to the Serotonin Surge food plan. Stay on it for a day or several days until the craving is under control and then return to phase 2. This is especially true if you find yourself craving snacks after dinner. Return immediately to an all-carbohydrate-and-vegetable dinner so that the after-dinner serotonin boost will keep you from snacking at night.

If you are on antidepressant medication and found that phase 1 diminished your cravings for carbs, you should find the carbohydrate in phase 2 adequate to keep them under control. If at any time your cravings return, go back to phase 1 until they are minimized.

Serotonin Balance Breakfast Guidelines

Breakfast is the same as in phase 1: one serving of protein, a starchy carbohydrate and fruit. (See pages 75 to 78 to review serving sizes.)

YOUR SEROTONIN BALANCE MEALS AND SNACKS

■ Breakfast: Protein, carbohydrate and a fruit or fruit juice. The fruit or fruit juice can be eaten at some other time of the day.

■ Snack: 1 hour before lunch

■ Lunch: Protein and vegetables

■ Snack: 3 or 4 hours after lunch

■ Dinner: Protein, carbohydrate and vegetables

Serotonin Balance Lunch Guidelines

Protein	Women (serving size)	Men (serving size)
Meat, poultry, seafood, fish, tofu, soya equivalent	90 g (3 oz)	145 g (5 oz)
Vegetables*	150–200 g (5½–7 oz) or more	150–200 g (5½–7 oz) or more

Beetroots and carrots should be limited to 200 g (7 oz)

Serotonin Balance Dinner Guidelines

Protein	Women (serving size)	Men (serving size)
Meat, poultry, seafood, fish, tofu, soya equivalent	60 g (2 oz)	115 g (4 oz)
Carbohydrate		
Basic grains and pulses, cooked: barley, bulgur wheat, chickpeas and other beans, couscous, buckwheat, lentils, millet, pasta, polenta, quinoa, rice, split peas	150 g (5½ oz)	230 g (8 oz)
Bread (30 g/1 oz slice)	3 slices	5 slices
Corn tortilla (15 cm/6 in)*	3	5
Flour tortilla (25 cm/10 in)	1	1½
Pitta, wholemeal or white 60 g (2 oz)	1½	2
Potato, sweet or white (raw weight)	230 g (8 oz)	340 g (12 oz)
Sweetcorn**	150 g (5½ oz)	250 g (9 oz)

Corn tortillas are low in calories. Use them as wraps and fill with rice and beans or other carbohydrate combinations.

**Sweetcorn makes a good dinner carb when combined with other starches like rice or couscous or when used as filling in a wrap.*

Vegetables	Women/Men (serving size)
Any combination of vegetables	150–200 g (5½–7 oz) or more
Carrots or beetroots*	Limit to 200 g (7 oz)**

These vegetables are restricted because they are dense.

**More than this will provide too many calories.*

Serotonin Balance Phase Recap

You must measure the amount of protein you are eating at dinner to ensure that you do not eat more than the recommended amount. If you prepare more protein than is allowed for dinner, save it for lunch the next day or freeze it for a quick meal later on. However, you don't have to eat protein for dinner. You can choose to eat only carbohydrate and vegetables for dinner at any time during the diet programme. Just follow the phase 1 dinner guidelines.

Sample Menus for the Serotonin Balance Phase

Recipes for the menu suggestions offered for each phase of the Good Mood Diet can be found in Chapter 14. Recipes are noted with an asterisk (*). For serving sizes, see the guidelines on pages 75 to 78 and on page 83.

Day 1 Serotonin Balance

Breakfast

Low-fat cottage cheese with pineapple

Low-fat muesli

Fresh strawberries

Snack, 1 hour before lunch

1 thick slice wholemeal bread

1 tablespoon whole-fruit jam

Lunch

Asian Seared Tuna Salad*

Snack, 3 hours after lunch

3 Snack-a-Jacks Chocolate Chip Rice Cakes

Dinner

Very Fast Beef and Broccoli with Rice*

Day 2 Serotonin Balance

Breakfast

English muffin

1 poached or scrambled egg

1 slice ham, very low fat

Melon

Snack, 1 hour before lunch

45 g (1½ oz) Kashi Honey 7-Grain cereal

Lunch

Sweet and Spicy Chicken*

Caribbean Salad*

Snack, 3 hours after lunch

40 g (1¼ oz) Japanese rice crackers

Dinner

Couscous with Lamb*

Sesame Mangetout*

Day 3 Serotonin Balance

Breakfast

Fat-free yogurt

Banana

Raisin toast

l teaspoon all-fruit jam

Snack, 1 hour before lunch

45 g (1½ oz) Fruit 'n' Fibre cereal

Lunch

Fish with Barbecue Sauce*

Mixed green salad with Chilli and Lime Dressing*

Snack, 3 hours after lunch

6 toasted coconut-covered marshmallows

Dinner

Polenta with Mushrooms and Meat*

Steamed vegetables with Italian Dressing*

PHASE 3: SEROTONIN CONTROL

Congratulations! You've arrived at the final 4 weeks of the diet, a time when losing weight, exercising and eating healthily is becoming second nature to you. If you reach your goal weight at the end of this phase, or wish to maintain your weight loss before losing more, you'll move to the maintenance phase (see Chapter 11). If you wish to continue losing weight, stay on the Serotonin Control phase until you reach your goal.

The objective of this final part of the programme is to help you keep losing weight while preparing you for the maintenance phase of the Good Mood Diet. To do this, your snacking will be limited to only once a day, in the late afternoon.

During this final phase, you can increase the variety of your snacks. Though the portion sizes have been decreased because your body needs less carbohydrate to boost serotonin, your snacks must continue to be high in carbohydrate and low in protein and fat.

YOUR SEROTONIN CONTROL MEALS AND SNACK

- Breakfast: Protein, carbohydrate and fruit or fruit juice. The fruit or fruit juice can be eaten at some other time of the day.
- Lunch: Protein and vegetables
- Snack: 3 to 4 hours after lunch
- Dinner: Protein, carbohydrate and vegetables

If at any time you feel that your appetite is not being controlled by eating only one snack a day or by the reduced portion size of the afternoon snack, you may return to the snack portion sizes and frequencies of the earlier phases of the diet plan.

In Serotonin Control, the meal guidelines are the same as for Phase 2. You will be eating protein, carbohydrate and fruit for breakfast; protein and vegetables for lunch; and protein, carbohydrate and vegetables for dinner.

Serotonin Control Breakfast Guidelines

Breakfast is the same as in phases 1 and 2: one serving of protein, a starchy carbohydrate and fruit. (See pages 75 to 76 to review serving sizes.)

Serotonin Control Lunch Guidelines

Lunch remains the same as in phase 2, consisting of protein and vegetables. Protein servings are 90 g (3 oz) for women and 145 g (5 oz) for men. Protein choices can include meat, poultry, fish, seafood, tofu or soya equivalent.

Both women and men should continue to eat 150–200 g (5½–7 oz) or more of vegetables, as noted on page 77, at lunch.

Serotonin Control Dinner Guidelines

Protein servings remain the same as they were in phase 2: 60 g (2 oz) for women and 115 g (4 oz) for men. Choices include meat, poultry, fish, seafood, tofu or soya equivalent.

Likewise, carbohydrate serving sizes remain the same in this phase. See pages 84 and 85 for a refresher on servings.

Both men and women should continue to eat 150–200 g (5½–7 oz) of vegetables, as noted on pages 77 to 78.

Serotonin Control Phase Recap

Pay attention to how much you are eating. During this part of the diet, failure to lose weight is often due to too-large portion sizes.

If you do not feel full after lunch, add a before-lunch carbohydrate snack. Use phase 1 and 2 snack portion sizes.

If you do not feel satisfied after dinner, add a mid-evening snack. Use phase 1 and 2 snack portion sizes.

Continue to restrict fat calories both in meals and in snacks.

If at any time you feel your control over your eating is at risk – for example during the days following holidays or during other stressful times – go back to phase 1 until your appetite is tamed once again.

Sample Menus for the Serotonin Control Phase

Recipes for the menu suggestions offered for each phase of the diet can be found in Chapter 14. Recipes are noted with an asterisk (*). For serving sizes, see the guidelines on pages 75 to 78 and page 83.

Day 1 Serotonin Control

Breakfast

Wholemeal toast

Low-fat ricotta cheese

Smoked salmon

Tomato

Red onion, thinly sliced, and capers (optional)

Lunch

Beef Stir-Fry*

Sliced pear

Snack, 3 hours after lunch

2 Jaffa Cakes

Dinner

Chicken Soup in a Hurry*

Mixed green salad with dressing* of choice

Day 2 Serotonin Control

Breakfast

Natural or lemon fat-free or low-fat yogurt

Strawberries, melon or blueberries

Low-fat muesli

Lunch

Prawn and Fennel Stir-Fry*

Mixed green salad with dressing of choice*

Snack, 3 hours after lunch

1 Skinny Cow Chocolate Fudge Stick

Dinner

Corn Burritos*

Steamed courgette

Baby carrots

Day 3 Serotonin Control

Breakfast

Rye bread, toasted

1 wedge Laughing Cow low-fat cheese

1 slice ham, very lean

½ grapefruit

Lunch

Asian Chicken Wrap*

Steamed broccoli with Japanese Dressing*

Baked apple drizzled with honey

Snack, 3 hours after lunch

15 g (½ oz) air-popped or microwave popcorn

Dinner

Pasta Shells with Smoked Salmon*

Roasted Asparagus with Vinaigrette*

Orange sorbet and fresh orange slices

FREQUENTLY ASKED QUESTIONS

What if my breakfast choices are limited and I can't get enough protein at breakfast?

You may be getting small amounts of protein from a couple of sources that you are overlooking. For example, milk added to coffee or tea, cheese spread added to your toast, or a small pot of yogurt all contribute protein to breakfast.

Whenever you don't eat enough protein at breakfast because of limited food choices, be sure to increase your serving of protein at lunch by 30–60 g (1–2 oz).

I noticed that there is very little fat in this diet. Don't we need a lot of fat to feel full? And isn't fat part of a healthy diet?

There are two reasons for the low-fat emphasis in the diet plan. The first is to eliminate extra calories. The second is to ensure that there is no delay in producing the serotonin response after you eat a carbohydrate meal or snack. The serotonin will make you feel full and satisfied without eating large quantities of fat.

Fat-free dairy products save you calories and unnecessary fat. However, their taste and texture vary. Experiment until you find a brand you like. If you really cannot tolerate skimmed milk but will drink semi-skimmed milk, then do so. It is better for you to have this excellent source of calcium in your diet than to avoid it totally because of a few extra calories.

Up to 1 tablespoon per serving of a high-fat cooking ingredient, such as oil or butter, or a flavour aid, such as cheese, crumbled bacon, crushed nuts, avocado, salad dressing or mayonnaise, are allowed in any one meal per day. Throughout all three phases, these fats work best for preparing dinner – but their use is at your discretion. Olive oil, rapeseed oil, nuts and avocados are among the healthiest fats, so choose these whenever possible. You will also get the health benefits of fish oils if you choose fatty fishes as your protein source.

I go to sleep very early. Do I have to stay awake to eat the phase 1 evening snack?

No, you don't. Just be sure to eat your other two snacks.

I buy all of my bread from the bakers. How much should I eat?

Buy bread shaped like a sandwich loaf and ask that it be sliced for you (each piece's size should be comparable to packaged, presliced bread). For a phase 1 dinner, figure on 3 slices for women and 4 slices for men. For a phase 2 or 3 dinner, figure on 2 slices for women and 3 slices for men.

I want to lose the weight I gained during my pregnancy, but I'm breast-feeding. Is it okay for me to be on the diet? Will it affect my milk?

You should consult with your doctor or your child's paediatrician before beginning any weight-loss programme. Remember that giving your baby adequate nutrition is more important than losing weight. However, if you eat wholesome and nutrient-packed foods, losing 0.5 kg (1 lb) a week is perfectly safe for you and your baby.

If you get your doctor's okay, use men's portions throughout the diet and eat an additional 60 g (2 oz) of protein daily. This will ensure that your milk production is not compromised and that your own and your child's nutritional requirements are being met.

I really like spicy foods. Can I use condiments?

You can add spices, herbs, hot sauces, chilli peppers and all kinds of fat-free and low-fat condiments to perk up your taste buds. Hot sauces, including Asian, Worcestershire and Tabasco, in addition to hoisin sauce, mustard, pickles, relish, horseradish, ketchup and chutney enliven all kinds of dishes.

Don't overlook beef, chicken, fish and vegetable stock. Cooking vegetables in a small amount of stock adds flavour without adding calories. Look for low-sodium varieties. Adding a squeeze of lemon juice to chicken stock increases the flavour of the stock and the vegetables.

I didn't see any alcohol in the menu suggestions. Did you forget to include it?

We did not forget. Alcohol adds unnecessary calories to your daily intake, and with all the carbohydrate in the diet, you will be feeling very relaxed without it. However, in phases 1 and 2, if it is necessary for you to drink (if, for example, you must make a toast or you must sample a special wine), limit your consumption to a sip or two or stick with one wine spritzer.

In phase 3 you can add a very moderate amount of alcohol since you are eliminating one of the snacks. Do not drink more than 1 glass of wine or 1 cocktail (and avoid any made with lots of cream). Be careful; drinking erodes eating control.

I started the Good Mood Diet in the summer and really did not crave carbohydrates. But now I am at the end of the diet and it is mid-autumn and my cravings are awful. What should I do?

You may be suffering from seasonal affective disorder, or SAD. As the days become darker, people feel their moods and appetite changing. Switch back to the Serotonin Balance phase until spring. This will allow you to control your cravings without risking weight gain. If you feel that two snacks a day are not enough during the darkest days of the year, add a third snack at night, as described for the Serotonin Surge phase.

I did all right on the Good Mood Diet until my mother-in-law was placed in a nursing home. Now I am so busy and upset that I cannot follow it. What should I do?

If you want to decrease your stress and control your eating under these difficult circumstances, make sure your serotonin levels are boosted. Stopping the diet may worsen the stress and make you likely to overeat and gain weight. If you don't have time to cook, choose foods that are fast and simple to prepare. Do not stop snacking on serotonin-boosting carbohydrate foods. It is extremely important that you maintain your serotonin levels so that you have the calmness and concentration to cope.

Also try to find a few minutes each day for yourself. Take a short walk, meditate, read a book or listen to music you enjoy. You must take care of yourself if you are to take care of others.

I have a teenage daughter, almost 15, who wants to follow the Good Mood Diet. Can she do it along with me?

Yes, with certain conditions. Teenagers typically skip breakfast, eat a nutritionally disastrous lunch, and are starved when they get home from school. If your teenager will not take a lunch to school, see if she will at least eat a protein bar. Leave salad and some vegetables for her to munch on, along with a carbohydrate snack, when she comes home. If she stays up late to do homework or text her friends, give her an evening carbohydrate snack as well. Also, to be safe, skip the Serotonin Surge phase and start with the Serotonin Balance phase. That way you will know that she is eating protein at dinner. And, of course, check with her doctor before she starts the diet.

Must I eat brown rice, brown pasta and so on, or can I have starchy foods made from refined flour?

Wholegrain foods have more fibre and nutrients than refined foods do. However, although it is important to eat such foods you do not need to *avoid* eating refined flour. Try to aim for a 50:50 balance to begin with; if you develop a taste for whole grains by all means increase the ration.

I like to sleep late on Sundays. When should I eat breakfast and my morning snack?

You can skip your morning snack as well as breakfast, but drink or eat your fruit. Then make your first meal large enough to include the protein and carbohydrate you normally would be eating for breakfast and lunch. Avoid high-fat foods like eggs Benedict, bacon, sausage and scrambled eggs dripping with butter. A three- or four-egg-white omelette with mushrooms, onions, tomatoes, spinach and a tiny bit of grated cheese is a good option. Prepare it with minimal oil. Have your first snack about 3 hours later, which will probably be around 3 or 4 p.m. Then eat supper about an hour or 2 after that. If you feel the need to eat something in mid-evening, have your second snack then.

What if I want to eat more than the recommended amount of chicken or another meat for dinner? Will I lose less weight if I do?

To keep the calories the same, you would have to decrease your dinner carbohydrate portion by one third or more. We have found that when our clients do this, they often find themselves craving something sweet soon after the meal is over. If you find yourself feeling full but not satisfied an hour or so after dinner, you did not have enough carbohydrate at dinner. So return to the guidelines. However, if you are satisfied and are content not to eat anything until breakfast the next day, you can increase your protein at dinner.

I love beans, like the baked kind, but I really feel bloated and uncomfortable afterwards. Should I not eat them at all?

Don't avoid them entirely. Rinse canned beans well and eat them in small quantities. Add a few tablespoons of beans to a rice dish or a tablespoon to your baked potato. When your body adjusts to these small servings, start increasing the size.

You can also try Beano, a natural enzyme product available in tablet and liquid forms. When taken with food, it helps your body digest beans as well as other 'gassy' foods such as broccoli, cabbage and onions.

Can I have stock made with meat for dinner in phase 1? I have a great recipe for chicken vegetable-rice soup.

Yes, as long as the rice and vegetables are the main component of the meal. When you get to phases 2 and 3, you can eat the meat in the stock or soup. Bean soup with ham, chicken and noodle soup, and beef and vegetable soup are all good phase 2 or 3 dinners.

How does lasagne fit into your diet plan?

While other pasta dishes do fit, lasagne doesn't. The cheeses traditionally found in the dish add too many calories, and the meat and sausage in the sauce add too much protein and fat. Some vegetarian lasagnes layer spinach rather than cheese between the noodles and use a meatless sauce. If you can make or order lasagne containing mostly vegetables and a small amount of a low-fat cheese such as low-fat ricotta, then you can have it for dinner.

CHAPTER SEVEN

Change Your Body

For many people, the thought of exercising brings up a host of reactions. Some of the most common ones we hear include:

- I hate it.
- I don't have time.
- I already exercise, but I'm not losing weight.

If you've ever made such excuses – or come up with others – ask yourself what you like less: exercising or being overweight.

You may never love exercise, but you can learn to love what exercise can do for you.

FACE THE FACTS

There is no getting around it. Exercise is a crucial component of losing weight and keeping it off. The reasons are straightforward.

Exercise will help you slim down because it burns calories.

As you age, your fat-to-muscle ratio increases. Exercise, particularly activities that force you to use muscles against resistance to build strength, such as walking up hills or weight training, replaces fat with muscle so you can reverse this process.

Building muscle burns calories. With more muscle mass, you appear more fit and toned.

Regular physical activity also allows dietary glucose that has entered the bloodstream to be converted to usable energy rather than stored as fat.

Regular exercise, specifically with strength training, will change your body, making it taut and firm.

A study of over 700 people who lost at least 13.5 kg (30 lb) and kept it off for at least a year stated, 'Nearly every participant used diet and exercise to initially lose weight, and nearly every subject is currently using diet and exercise to maintain his/her weight loss.'[1]

Also, a recent study conducted at the Mayo Clinic in Minnesota, USA, showed that lean people spent less time throughout the day sitting than obese people did.[2] In this study, lean people walked, stood up and moved around much more than their sedentary counterparts. The study showed that obese subjects sat 152 minutes more a day – more than 2½ hours more – than slimmer subjects did. That translated into 350 fewer calories burned by the heavier subjects. The conclusion was that activity throughout the day adds up. This kind of increased daily activity can help you lose weight. To drop 0.5 kg (1 lb) of body fat, you need to expend 3,500 calories. Your body doesn't care how you do it – even fidgeting works in your favour.

You might not think of a lot of daily activities as weight-loss helpers. Activities like window washing, stair climbing, running around with your kids, pushing a pram, raking leaves, painting, carrying heavy objects such as shopping bags, gardening, taking the stairs instead of the lift, walking instead of driving, pacing while on the phone and vacuuming the house all add up.

Here's a simple way to monitor how 'far' you are going. Wear a pedometer and aim for 10,000 steps a day, which roughly translates into walking 5 miles. This small inexpensive gadget slips onto your clothing at your hip and tracks your daily movements.

Physical activity does all kinds of other good things for your body and your mind. Exercise builds stamina and strength. It can reduce the risk of cardiovascular disease (heart attack, stroke and high blood pressure), diabetes, back pain and osteoporosis. It can elevate mood, make you feel good about yourself, alleviate anxiety and help with stress management. It can also improve sleep and offer rewarding challenges while helping you form new skills and add fun to your life.

Exercise can also help to alleviate depression, according to a study that appeared in the *Journal of Preventive Medicine*. The amount of recommended exercise – a half hour a day, 6 days a week – resulted in a significant reduction of symptoms in a group of depressed patients. Even more remarkable, the exercise benefit was similar to outcomes experienced when patients took antidepressant medication.[3]

IF YOU ALREADY EXERCISE

But maybe you exercise and you're still overweight. If that is the case, your body may have become very efficient at doing your current workout. That means you are burning fewer calories and not building new muscles. Therefore, your body needs to work harder.

You may have to increase the frequency of your exercise, vary the activities you do to work a variety of muscles, enhance the intensity of what you do or spend more time exercising.

The most efficient way to make exercise more effective is to add strength training. For instance, hold hand weights when you do lunges, do your situps slowly, push yourself harder in Pilates class, or raise the elevation on the treadmill. When your muscles are worked hard, your body burns fat for energy.

If you want to lose weight, it isn't enough to just go for a walk a couple of times a week; you need to take the stairs instead of the lift, park your car a good distance from your destination, and get up every hour or so from your computer and move around. These movements will burn some extra calories, improve your cardiovascular health by getting the blood pumping regularly throughout the day, and keep you from getting stiff – but they are not enough if you want to really lose weight.

We're not suggesting that you run marathons or train for an Ironman competition. However, we do recommend what works.

ALL YOU NEED TO DO

The ideal blend of exercise is aerobic plus strength training, preferably achieved by performing a variety of activities. This combination burns more fat than aerobic exercise alone. This is especially important for women, since doing aerobic exercise alone burns only a minimal amount of their body fat.

If you perform only non-resistance aerobic activity (like jogging) and your hunger increases, you may overeat and the extra calories will be stored as fat with no opportunity for your body to replace that fat with muscle. On the other hand, if you only do non-aerobic exercise, you'll only be able to eat a very low number of calories (less than 1,200) in order to take in fewer calories than are being expended. On such a low-calorie diet, not only is it difficult to get all the essential nutrients, but you can also feel extremely hungry and launch your body into a starvation state – which slows down your body's metabolism. Thus, without aerobic activity, even if you consume few calories, weight loss is difficult.

Cross-training, defined as doing several different forms of exercise, is our preferred type of workout because it consistently uses different muscles so more calories are burned. Variety is important because muscles are highly adaptable. If you do not vary your exercise regime, your muscles will become efficient and burn fewer calories than if you mixed your physical activities. In addition, change prevents overuse injury and alleviates boredom.

Once you reach your goal weight, the amount of exercise you take can be scaled back slightly to maintain your new size. Hopefully, the many other benefits of physical activity, in addition to maintaining weight loss, will keep you exercising even when your goal weight is reached.

Establishing a regular exercise regime takes time. That's why we developed a 12-week programme. We found that it takes around 4 weeks to break a pattern of not exercising and 8 more weeks to start establishing a new habit. Our 12-week guide in Chapter 9 will help you reinforce your new habits.

You need to make a commitment you can stick with and focus on the process, not the end result. Starting an exercise plan and following through with it is essential for weight loss. In fact, the planning and follow-through are often more important than the particular physical activity you choose to do.

We recommend consulting your doctor before starting an exercise programme. And keep in mind that if after you begin your programme you feel any pain or discomfort beyond mild muscle achiness, you must let your doctor know about it.

THE REQUIREMENTS

Half an hour a day pushes the weight away. That's only 3½ hours a week – not much, considering that a week has 168 hours – in addition to moving around during the day as much as possible.

If you currently exercise infrequently or not at all, you will gradually build up to this weekly time commitment. After that, you'll increase the intensity of your activities.

For those of you who exercise now or who want an additional challenge, the duration, frequency and intensity of your regime can be increased as long as you don't risk injury to yourself. Listen to your body.

Our weekly prescription is simple:

- Four sessions of aerobic activity in the fat-burning zone (see below) that last a minimum of 30 minutes each.
- Three sessions of strength training that exhaust your muscles and last a minimum of 30 minutes each.

If you don't want to exercise every day, you can put together any combination of aerobic and strength training. For example, on 3 days you can do both aerobic activity and strength training and on the 4th day perform only aerobic exercise. However, we do strongly recommend that you continue to increase your regular movements (like taking the stairs or parking further away) each day.

As long as you don't have a medical limitation like asthma or a heart condition, you need to increase your heart rate to get into the aerobic fat-burning zone specific for your age. In the aerobic fat-burning zone, your body works hard enough to burn fat for energy. To find your fat-burning zone, complete the calculation below.

$$\text{Your fat-burning zone} = (220 - \text{your age}) \times 0.75$$

We strongly recommend using a heart-rate monitor when you do aerobic exercise. It will tell you whether you are working hard enough. If you don't have one, you'll know that you are exercising hard enough if you cannot comfortably carry on a full conversation. So it's worth keeping quiet when you're in that fat-burning exercise zone!

Remember: every body is different. It's up to you to determine the exact amount and type of exercise you need to lose weight and keep it off. As long as you are mindful of injury prevention and your health limitations, you can gradually increase the intensity of your activities and, if your schedule permits, the amount of time you spend doing them. Begin slowly and build up. Every day is different. You know yourself. Pace yourself accordingly.

The point is this: exercise works. Our successful clients do it regularly. Our clients who do not exercise regularly struggle to lose weight and keep it off. No matter what activity you choose to do, the best exercise is one that is done. (Just remember to wear good exercise shoes. Your feet will thank you.)

AEROBIC ACTIVITIES

Aerobic exercise is any continuous, rhythmic activity that utilizes large muscle groups.

Types

Aerobic activities include power walking, hill walking, running, jogging, ice skating, dancing (belly, Latin, modern, tap, folk, ballroom), tennis, skiing, cycling, circuit training with no more than 30 seconds of rest between exercises, indoor aerobic machines (treadmill, elliptical trainer, stationary bike, step climber, cross-country ski machine, rowing machine), swimming, canoeing, skipping, volleyball, water aerobics, aerobics classes, and using a hula hoop.

Some aerobic activities, such as swimming, cycling uphill and kickboxing, also provide strength training because the body has to work against a force such as water, gravity or a punch bag.

Benefits

Aerobic activities reduce the risk of heart disease, burn calories and improve psychological well-being.

Weekly Prescription

Do four 30-minute sessions or a total of 2 hours spread over the week. If an aerobic activity involves a significant strength-training component, count one half of that activity as aerobic exercise and the other as strength training.

If you are reluctant to increase the intensity on an indoor aerobic machine, give yourself a 3-minute challenge. Then resume your usual intensity. Then, try the challenge for 5 minutes. You soon may find the confidence to do it for even longer.

STRENGTH TRAINING AND CORE CONDITIONING

Strength training includes any activity that challenges your muscles to work against a force. That force could be a heavy object, maintaining your body in a certain position, or engaging muscles to control how you move. Putting a muscle to work causes microscopic damage to the muscle fibres, which leads to the repairing and building up of the muscle, thus making it stronger. Strength training includes core conditioning, which refers to the strengthening of central muscle groups, such as the abdominal and back muscles.

Types

Strength workouts include circuit weight training, resistance-band exercises, free-weight training, callisthenics (squats, lunges, abdominal crunches, press-ups), swimming, water aerobics, step aerobics, boxing or kickboxing, cycling uphill, strenuous hill walking, Pilates, yoga (especially the vigorous styles), balance-ball exercises, ballet and tai chi.

Benefits

Strength training builds and strengthens muscles, toning them so you look better. Consequently, your confidence is increased (with the possible added side effect of feeling sexier). Strength training also boosts body awareness, which can be a tool for stress management, and improves posture, which increases control of movements. This is important not only for gracefulness but also for injury prevention.

Weekly Prescription

Do three sessions lasting 30 minutes each. An hour of strength training that includes aerobic activity counts as 30 minutes of aerobic activity and 30 minutes of strength training. During each session, it is best to engage in a few focused exercises or movements so you can fully challenge and exhaust a particular muscle group. This is more effective than trying to quickly get through as many different exercises as possible.

If you use free weights, choose a weight heavy enough for each exercise set so that by the end of 10 to 12 repetitions you cannot do even 1 more (until the next set). Do each repetition slowly, without using momentum to get you through the range of motion. Concentrate on the muscle or muscles being worked, and aim for two or three sets. Ladies, don't fear 'bulking up'. Remember, weight training will make you look leaner because the increasing muscle mass will replace fat, which takes up more room than muscle. How much you bulk up is partly genetic, and female bodybuilders do so by using very high weights and performing many repetitions. However, if after a few months of weight training you notice your muscles becoming too big for your taste, cut down on the weight you're lifting and do 15 to 18 repetitions per set instead of 10 to 12.

STRETCHING

Stretching should complement your aerobic and strength training. Do a variety of stretches to increase flexibility and involve as many muscles and joints as possible. Perform enough of them so that you progressively become more flexible.

Types

You can learn new stretches from books, at a stretch class, or from a video or television programme.

Benefits

Stretching prevents injury, increases the range and variety of movements, lessens stiffness in joints and improves both exercise performance and the quality of movement throughout daily activities.

Weekly Prescription

Spend at least 5 to 10 minutes stretching every day, and more if you can. In those few minutes, you can stretch out commonly tight areas such as the neck, shoulders, lower back, hips, hamstrings and calves. Spending even more time can deepen the stretches and allow you to focus on other areas that might need relaxing.

Whenever you stretch, make sure you ease into it gently and keep your breathing natural – that is, don't strain or hold your breath. Natural breathing will allow you to go deeper into the stretch and avoid injury.

Stretching should always be done for at least 5 minutes after exercise when the muscles are warmed up and looser. Increased flexibility and lessened muscle soreness will be your rewards.

THE BEST EXERCISE FOR YOU

You know what motivates you, what your constraints are, what best fits into your schedule and what you will realistically do. Check the exercise solutions below to help resolve your workout problems.

You have no time Exercise at high intensity to use the time you have efficiently and effectively. You can do it in brief sessions throughout the day, such as walking up and down stairs for 10 minutes or doing a couple of weight-training activities for 5 minutes at a time. Put exercise on your calendar, dropping another obligation if necessary. You can work out with a morning TV exercise programme. Check your local TV listings for body-toning, yoga, stretch, step aerobics or other such fitness programmes you can follow in the convenience of your home. You can record these programmes to fit them into your schedule. Some digital cable and satellite TV packages come with workout programmes

IF YOU FEEL TIRED

If fatigue (such as that caused by medication or lack of sleep) makes exercising initially seem daunting, start by blocking off up to 30 minutes of time on your calendar and simply commit to challenging your body in some way. Do not get overly concerned by what you can or cannot do. Instead, focus on being active and doing some form of exercise. Put on your exercise clothes and shoes to get in the mood. Take a walk, go to the gym or an exercise class, get a workout friend to encourage you, or follow an exercise DVD. Be gentle with yourself in terms of what you can and cannot do and know that you will only improve over time – maybe even faster than you think. Remember: exercising may make you sleep better, giving you more energy for other activities.

that you can watch at any time, and those of you who own MP3 players can download exercise programmes.

You hate exercising Be creative about your choice. Join a dance class or train for a race to support a charity. Go for long walks with a friend, chase your kids around the garden or park, or walk to work.

You need a challenge Sign up for a 5-K running race and record your time as you train. Run with someone who is faster than you or play tennis with someone who is better than you. Take up horse riding, sign up for swimming lessons or book an adventure such as a cycling trip so you'll be forced to get in shape.

You hate clutter A compact step climber, a set of hand weights, a yoga mat and aerobics videos, like one that teaches kickboxing, don't take up much space. Garages are full of unused exercise equipment. If you want to buy free weights, treadmills or home-gym machines check ads in local papers and even eBay. The bargains you'll find will pay you back big time.

You need peer pressure Join an exercise class with a friend, hire a trainer or do a group workout session. If you are seeking more social situations, exercise classes offer the opportunity to meet people. You already share something in common, which can lessen the awkwardness of speaking to someone new.

Lots of people want to exercise with someone they know. If this is an incentive to you, ask your friends what kinds of workouts they do or are interested in doing.

You want a holistic exercise experience Choose yoga or Pilates plus an outdoor aerobic activity like hill walking or power walking.

You need a routine to get anything done Exercise at the same time every day – no matter what activity you choose.

You can't afford to join a gym or buy exercise equipment There are plenty of free or low-cost activities: follow city or countryside trails, swim at a local authority swimming pool or why not join the growing number of people who do outdoor tai chi classes. Alternatively, just a little money will buy a weight-training book or an exercise DVD, hand weights and resistance bands.

Do you like to walk? Terrific. Wear comfortable shoes and stride at a brisk pace. If you can, try to get from one errand to another on foot. When you are at work, you can use part of your lunch break to walk laps around the vicinity of your office.

You hate monotony If you are an executive, bring a small treadmill into your office. Get on it whenever you need a break. Some people find that exercise clears the mind, so time spent using the treadmill may spark some very creative solutions. Read a magazine, listen to a book on tape, or watch TV as you pedal on an exercise bike.

You don't want to exercise with others If being overweight makes you feel uncomfortable about exercising among others, find an environment in which you feel at ease. If that's your living room, perfect. Or visit a few gyms to see if the clientele shares your fitness level. You might feel at home there, too.

DVDs might be just the thing. To get started, go to the library or surf the Internet and pick a few that appeal to you. If you haven't exercised in a while, start with a gentle beginner's programme. A friend might have a recommendation.

Exercise can help reduce stress. Often anxiety shows itself in a tensing of the muscles; anger can do the same. Vigorous activity can loosen your muscles so they are no longer tight. Yoga is particularly good for this because it stretches and relaxes different muscles simultaneously. Exercise forces you to focus on your breathing and what you are doing, thereby distracting you from your problems.

USE THE MOTIVATION THAT WORKS FOR YOU

A lot of clients tell us that it takes a momentous event to push them to exercise. Sometimes it's a joyous occasion, like a wedding or a long-anticipated holiday. The person wants to look great and is willing to do whatever is necessary, particularly for the short-term.

But the more frightening incidents can exert a greater influence. A parent gets sick, and suddenly genetics becomes a concern. A friend dies, and all at once health issues that might not have been considered become very important. Or a child has a weight problem and the parent realizes that setting an example is crucial. Fear is a powerful motivator, especially for getting started.

On the other hand, many clients find that receiving compliments on how terrific they look keeps them focused once they start exercising.

For example, one of our clients, a 43-year-old mother of a 6-year-old, consistently went to a dance class. She related that the whole class, along with the teacher, commented on her shrinking size practically every week. It was a huge ego boost that always kept her coming back for more.

Once you start, it's very likely that you will motivate yourself. If you slip and fall off the exercise bandwagon, you will start to miss it. Your body will give you lots of hard-to-ignore symptoms. You'll be stiffer, have trouble sleeping, feel less energetic and start eating more.

Tip: Get a headset phone and move around, stretch or do squats while you chat. Or do sit-ups while you watch TV.

SEE WHAT IS POSSIBLE

Jessica, a 36-year-old software marketing director and self-proclaimed perfectionist, often stayed at work until 7 or 8 p.m. Fed up with being unfit and overweight, she realized that, like some of her colleagues who left work with their gym bags, perhaps her work would not suffer if she went to a weekly 6 p.m. aerobics class. She found that not only did her work not suffer, she felt more energetic the day after her class. Eventually Jessica added a 6 p.m. body-conditioning class. The scheduled commitments forced her to work more efficiently and delegate more, because she had an exercise appointment to go to at the end of the day.

George and Linda, an overweight couple in their forties who decided to lose weight together, started to power walk. Every Saturday and Sunday, as well as a couple of weeknights after dinner, they laced up their walking shoes and took a brisk half-hour walk around their town. Not only did they get their exercise, they also had time together without distractions because of their 'no mobile phone' rule.

Michael, 41, who excelled at planning the finances of his clients, finally adapted this skill for himself. He bought a planner specifically for daily and weekly planning and used it to motivate him to exercise. When he wrote 'go to gym' and 'take walk' in it, the commitment became real and he was able to follow through.

Sal, a 66-year-old retired stonemason, had gained over 22.5 kg (50 lb) that he wanted to lose. Recently divorced, he desired a new social life. Because years of working with heavy materials had put a strain on all of his joints, we helped him find an experienced yoga instructor for private at-home sessions. In addition, we instructed him to walk on the grounds of a nearby golf course, instead of on the streets, for brief periods several times a day. Eventually, he attended group yoga classes filled with others his age. The women in the class inspired him to keep doing yoga; additionally, he found new walking companions and a renewed social life.

Doris was doing great with her exercise and diet programme and she wanted her husband, who sat behind a desk all day and on the sofa the rest of the time, to do the same. Knowing him well, she used potential embarrassment as a tool. They had talked for years about doing a walking tour of the English lakes. When Doris retired from her job as a schoolteacher, she booked a 2-week trip to the lakes for the following summer. Her husband, knowing that she would outwalk him, finally began to get in shape.

Josh, who at 30 still carried the 9 kg (20 lb) he had gained in his first year at university, made a bet with his sister. Whoever lost the weight in 4 months would win a paid weekend away with their spouse. He took up running and won the bet in 3 months.

Kate, a serial dieter, started losing the 18 kg (40 lb) she had gained. A 29-year-old stay-at-home mum, she hired a personal trainer to come to her house. But when her husband saw the trainer he balked. The money didn't bother him, but the trainer's sculpted physique and good looks did. Kate insisted, her husband resisted, and finally they reached a compromise. If a couple of Kate's friends joined her, then her husband wouldn't have a problem with the trainer. Kate agreed and recruited a couple of girlfriends to work out with her. Everyone won.

After you decide on an exercise or sport you like and do it for a while, you may be ready for something new. Trial and error is a sane way to approach exercise. If you like it, do it. If you don't, forget it.

Tip: If you can, get a dog – preferably one that is a fast walker. You'll be forced to take rapid walks, too.

THE LAMEST EXCUSES NOT TO EXERCISE

Over the years we've heard some astonishing excuses from clients for not exercising. We would like to share our all-time favourites.

It's a full moon.

My trainers need replacing.

I've been driving around all day doing errands.

I forgot my socks.

I had to wait for a delivery man.

I'm having a bad hair day.

There's an eclipse.

I couldn't find a parking space near the gym.

I just had a pedicure and/or manicure.

It's a holiday.

The magazines at the gym are out-of-date.

My dog is too tired to walk.

My horoscope said not to exercise.

It's my birthday.

I feel fat.

THE SEASONAL MOTIVATION EFFECT

In many parts of the world, winter, with its short days and long nights, can turn even the best-intentioned exerciser into a world-class couch potato. Prolonged periods of rainy weather can do the same. The lack of exposure to adequate sunlight is to blame.

How do you exercise when you can't even get off the sofa? The solution is to readjust your expectations of what you should do and make your environment as conducive to exercise as possible.

On dark, cold or wet days, you may need to reduce the intensity of your exercise regime, making it a way to not gain weight until the sunlight comes back. You can still get health benefits from more gentle activities. So:

- Tone down the resistance (intensity) on an aerobic machine
- Walk rather than run
- Reduce the resistance intensity of your weight training
- Join a gentle yoga or stretch class

Many people find that donning weather-appropriate clothing and taking a brisk walk in the cold, wind or rain can be energizing. If that doesn't appeal to you at all, perhaps walking around a heated shopping centre or a temperature-controlled museum will.

Health clubs, with their bright lights and music, can elevate mood. If your exercise machine sits in a dark place, it can depress you and decrease your willingness to exercise. For the winter, at least, join a club on a monthly basis. Find a welcoming gym with easy parking if you can't walk to it, or one near public transport.

You might also consider taking an adult education class to learn how to tango or do some other dance. It's good exercise – and you will wow everyone at the next wedding you go to.

Find something you can do in any season or vary your activity depending on the season. Maybe you like to cycle but bad weather sometimes prevents you from doing so. A second-hand treadmill or bicycle isn't expensive but remember: you can run or walk anytime. Just dress accordingly.

Respect your limitations and find the positives in what you can do rather than feeling bad about what you are not doing. Just be sure to return to your usual intensity once the sunlight, and your good mood and energy, return.

GIVE YOURSELF REWARDS

One of our clients shared her method for regular exercising. 'I've committed to going to a women-only gym 3 days a week. The convenience is fabulous: the place is literally around the corner from my flat. Also, the only 'equipment' I had to buy was a decent pair of trainers. I wear old shorts and T-shirts. The days I choose are up to me, which gives me flexibility. Sometimes I go on Saturday mornings, especially if I know that the week ahead will be busy. I always go in the morning for three reasons. First, I get it out of the way. Second, if the day doesn't turn out too well I know that I've accomplished one thing I wanted to do. Third, and most important, is that I get to eat breakfast and read a section of the paper afterward.'

One client scheduled a massage for the weekend when she had gone to the gym three times that week. Another looked forward to the time spent with a friend. Exercising together gave them a much-needed excuse to see each other. Still another found that competing against himself worked: 'I push myself to do more minutes on the elliptical trainer each time until I reach my goal.'

Another client, a woman in her seventies, had no problem following the diet plan but was very resistant to doing enough exercise. Despite her age – or perhaps because of it – she sported a gorgeously coifed head of expertly dyed blonde hair.

When asked why she wouldn't exercise she gave us the 'I'm really an old grey head' excuse.

Then we pointed out that it was obviously important to her to look as good as she could, and that if she exercised like a young blonde she would achieve it.

After that, exercise was never an issue.

FREQUENTLY ASKED QUESTIONS

I have a physical disability [or injury] that prevents me from exercising in the conventional sense. What can I do?

Work with a physiotherapist, doctor, qualified chiropractor or another trained and experienced professional who can help you devise a safe and effective exercise regime. Spend more time doing gentle exercise, and try swimming or yoga with an experienced teacher.

Do I have to breathe quickly? I don't feel comfortable doing it.

Start slowly and your breathing will get easier. If you have asthma, see your doctor for tips on optimum control.

Will exercise make me hungrier?

Not necessarily. For some, exercise actually suppresses appetite, but if you've increased your aerobic activity, you are burning more calories and your appetite may increase as a result. That's because when you burn up calories, you feel genuine hunger that will allow you to distinguish between a need to eat and an urge to eat.

Exercise also provides structure to the day. If you know you are going to exercise at a given time, you are more likely to time your meals rather than nibble throughout the day.

If I exercise a lot, will I finally get rid of my flabby belly?

Be realistic about the body proportions you were born with and realize that the more fit you are overall, the better you will look and feel no matter what the makeup of your body is. Resistance training can firm your abdominal muscles and reduce underarm 'wings', improving your natural physique.

Will I have to maintain for the rest of my life the same high level of exercise that helped me lose weight?

No. When you reach your goal weight you can start to reduce the amount you exercise, paying close attention to how much exercise you need to do to keep the weight off.

I'm breast-feeding. Can I follow the same exercise guidelines as everyone else?

Injury prevention is of utmost importance because your body went through enormous changes through pregnancy. At the same time, you may weigh more and be chronically sleep-deprived from frequent night-time feedings. Both can affect how you exercise, as can hormones that support lactation. Listen to your body. If you feel strain or sheer exhaustion, cut back. Movie stars may feel the pressure to be in 'perfect' shape 3 months after giving birth, but your goal is to get stronger and leaner and feel more positive about yourself at a pace that is right for you.

Now What Do I Do?

While you're on the Good Mood Diet you're also living your life. Business lunches, getting together with friends, going out for a meal with your family: all these activities must – and should – go on.

But when you dine away from home you still have to be aware of portion sizes and the fat content of food. Many of our clients travel constantly or hate cooking. Others keep schedules that cause them to eat all their meals at work and at catered lunches or dinners.

EATING IN RESTAURANTS

Knowing how much to eat when you're away from home can be challenging. In recent years, portion sizes have increased in restaurants, not just in fast food outlets. Assume that you will be served a portion larger than that recommended in any phase of the diet plan. For instance, if you order pasta as a main course you probably will be served 4 or more cups. Potatoes in steak houses usually weigh 12 to 16 ounces, which is OK for phase 1 but too big for phases 2 and 3. Fish, chicken, and beef main courses at dinnertime run between 8 and 10 ounces, and more at steak houses.

The only restaurant foods that do not exceed the diet's guidelines are vegetables. In fact, many restaurants do not bother serving vegetables with the main course. If they are served, they tend to be in very small quantities and often are swimming in copious amounts of butter or oil. This is also true of many salads and their heavy dressings.

Obviously you cannot march into a restaurant kitchen armed with a set of measuring scales and a ruler. But you can do several things to make sure you eat portions appropriate for weight loss.

Train your eye to recognize the amount of food you should eat
When you are at home, measure or weigh foods and teach yourself to recognize the appropriate portion size of rice, pasta or chicken. Then you can make an educated guess about how much of the meal you should eat when you dine out. If you share a protein main course or eat part of it and take the rest home for lunch or dinner the following day, figure a lunch portion is 170 g (6 oz) and a dinner portion is 230 g (8 oz). Divide accordingly.

Ask about the portion sizes If you tend to go to the same restaurant over and over again, ask the waiter to get the portion sizes from the chef. Every head chef knows precisely how much food goes on a plate because portion size is built into the financial structure and inventory control of the restaurant. You will usually get the same number of prawns or weight of chicken or rice each time you order. Don't feel that you have to explain why you need this information. No one has to know that you are on a diet.

Request that minimal or no oil be used in preparing your meal
This is a good way to avoid hidden fats. Restaurants and caterers rely on fats such as butter and olive oil to keep foods that may have been prepared hours beforehand tasting fresh.

Ask about preparation When ordering a new dish or visiting a new restaurant, always ask the waiter how it is prepared. There are always ingredients that are not included in the menu description.

Request food not on the menu If you don't see something on the menu that you want to eat, like a baked potato or an egg-white omelette, ask if that item is available. Often the food is in the kitchen, but not on the printed menu.

Call ahead There is nothing to prevent you calling a restaurant in advance if you are uncertain of what type of food they serve. You also can request ahead of time that foods be prepared in a certain way. To make sure he does not become seriously ill, one of our clients who has a severe food allergy calls ahead to inform the staff and then asks to see the chef when he arrives.

Your dessert of choice at all restaurants should be fruit. If you must taste another kind of dessert, limit yourself to a forkful of someone else's, but do not order one yourself. Drink a cup of coffee or tea while the desserts are passed around. If you feel tempted, use this time to go to the toilet so the desserts are finished by the time you return.

Fighting Hidden Fats

A side dish of rice at a restaurant serving American-style food may contain substantial amounts of butter or oil to keep it from drying out. If the choice at such a restaurant is between rice and a baked potato, opt for the potato. In contrast, rice at a Chinese restaurant (unless it is a fast-food place) won't contain fat. The rice is continually being made, kept warm in a cooker, and served.

It is not necessary to insist that restaurant food be defatted with a blowtorch, but do be alert. If you are uncertain about the fat content of a dish, ask. Many soups or sauces contain lots of cream, cheese or butter. Inquiring can help you avoid ordering something that is inappropriate for the Good Mood Diet.

RESTAURANT CHOICES

In response to clients' requests, we developed restaurant guidelines that make it easy to stick to the diet, regardless of what phase you are following.

Italian and Asian restaurants offer foods that are the most compatible with the diet plan. Indian and Mexican restaurants and steak houses require more care in finding suitable menu choices. Fast-food places fall somewhat short in meeting your diet needs, but you can still find diet-appropriate foods if you look hard.

Italian

Italian restaurants have a reputation for serving large portions of food loaded with oily sauces and cheese. But Italian restaurants also offer plenty of low-fat options you can choose to suit all phases of the diet.

Lunch, all phases: Roasted chicken with grilled vegetables; large mixed salad with grilled prawns; baked, steamed or roasted fish with sautéed spinach; seafood salad.

Dinner, phase 1: Any pasta without added cheese or cream sauce, such as pasta primavera or vegetable-filled tortellini. Bruschetta, bread, pizza with most of the cheese scraped off, and minestrone soup are also good options. Do not worry if the red sauce on your pasta has a meat base or small amounts of meat cooked in; the amount of protein is very small. Pasta and clams is also a good option since the sauce is usually white wine and clam stock and the clams are usually tiny. Add a large salad and a side order of a steamed vegetable to these dishes.

Dinner, phases 2 and 3: The same as for phase 1, plus roasted chicken, grilled fish, veal stew, veal marsala, veal in lemon sauce or grilled lean steak.

Avoid: Dipping bread in olive oil (doing so can add hundreds of additional calories), extra cheese, cream sauce, any cheese-stuffed pasta, breaded dishes like veal Parmesan, fried calamari, and pasta dripping in oil.

Chinese

Though many of us associate Chinese cuisine with fried rice and wontons, you can make numerous delicious choices in any phase of the diet. Best of all, using chopsticks prevents you from eating too much oil or sauce.

Lunch, all phases: Stir-fried chicken, tofu, shellfish, beef or pork (meats used in Chinese restaurants are very lean) with broccoli or other vegetables. Soups featuring fish, chicken, pork or beef are wonderful options as well.

Dinner, phase 1: Rice and any assortment of vegetables, particularly stir-fried or steamed green beans or broccoli (spinach and watercress absorb more oil); steamed vegetarian pot sticker dumplings; vegetarian moo shu (thin pancakes used to wrap chopped vegetables). If you are sharing the meal with others, eat the vegetable portion of any meat, fish or chicken dish they order (like prawn and black mushrooms). If there is leftover protein, take it home for lunch the next day.

Dinner, phases 2 and 3: Stir-fried meat, tofu or seafood with vegetables and steamed (not fried) rice; soups featuring fish, chicken, pork or beef with rice noodles. Do not worry about the sauces. Unless you are scooping up the food with a ladle, the extra calories added by the sauce will not interfere with your weight loss.

Avoid: Deep-fried and oil-laden foods such as crispy fried noodles dipped in sweet and sour sauce, noodles like lo mein (which are prepared with large amounts of oil to prevent them from sticking), spare ribs and fried prawns.

You can eat the fortune cookie.

Japanese

Japanese food typically is very low in fat, and usually many vegetable dishes are available, making it a great choice for all phases of the diet. Sushi makes a great take-away dinner, and sashimi can be eaten with vegetables for lunch. Be aware that seaweed is high in monosodium glutamate; if you are MSG-sensitive, avoid it.

Lunch, all phases: Sashimi or salmon, tofu or chicken teriyaki with steamed vegetables or seaweed salad; hot-pot soup featuring beef, chicken, seafood, egg or tofu; miso soup.

Dinner, phase 1: Vegetarian sushi, rice with sautéed vegetables, hot-pot soup featuring vegetables and rice or wheat noodles; steamed spinach; mixed green or seaweed salad (ask for dressing on the side); miso soup.

Dinner, phases 2 and 3: Sushi with seafood and vegetables; salmon, tofu or chicken teriyaki with rice and steamed vegetables; hot-pot soup featuring beef, chicken, seafood, tofu or egg and rice, wheat or soba noodles; miso soup.

Avoid: Tempura as a main dish, since it will be too high in calories. However, feel free to enjoy a couple of pieces of these batter-dipped fried vegetables.

Mexican

Enjoy as much salsa as you want. It is low in calories.

Lunch, all phases: Large salad with cucumber, tomato, pepper and onion, grilled chicken, grilled steak strips; roast chicken with steamed vegetables; prawns with vegetables. Avoid the restaurant tortillas, which tend to be high in fat.

Dinner, phase 1: Fajitas with vegetables and rice and a tortilla; large mixed green salad; kidney or black beans (not cooked in lard); black bean soup with tortillas.

Dinner, phases 2 and 3: Fajitas with stir-fried beef (it is very lean), chicken or prawns; large mixed green salad with grilled chicken or beef; chicken tortilla soup without tortilla chips, avocado, or added cheese; black bean soup with a side order of grilled chicken.

Avoid: Guacamole, soured cream, refried beans, dishes smothered in cheese, tortilla chips and the fried tortilla shells that salads often come in.

Indian

While Indian food can contain an enormous amount of oil or ghee (clarified butter), a number of choices do fit into the diet plan.

Lunch, all phases: Grilled or tandoori-cooked chicken or fish; mixed green salad; lentil or other bean soup without cream or coconut milk; mulligatawny soup

Dinner, phase 1: Vegetable and chickpea dishes with minimal ghee or oil accompanied by rice and raita (a yogurt-cucumber mixture); mixed salads and small portions of naan, or roti, chapati or paratha.

Dinner, phases 2 and 3: Tandoori chicken or fish accompanied by rice and grilled vegetables and raita; low-fat chicken or lentil stew with rice.

Avoid: Meats and vegetables prepared with large amounts of oil or cheese, curry dishes loaded with coconut milk and ghee, fried appetizers such as samosas, and other deep-fried foods like poori (bread).

Thai

Lunch, all phases: Stir-fried beef, chicken, seafood or tofu with vegetables; chicken or prawn satay (ask to have the peanut sauce on the side and use it sparingly); meat and seafood soups made without coconut milk.

Dinner, phase 1: Vegetarian pad thai; steamed or stir-fried vegetables with rice; vegetable soups made without coconut milk; fresh vegetarian spring rolls; green papaya salad.

Dinner, phases 2 and 3: Chicken or prawn satay (with minimal peanut sauce) and rice; stir-fried noodles with beef, prawn, chicken, tofu or egg; stir-fried beef, chicken, seafood or tofu with vegetables and steamed rice; green papaya salad.

Avoid: Fried spring rolls and wontons, curries and soups made with coconut milk, crispy fish, fried ice cream, and iced coffee or tea made with condensed milk.

Steak Houses

Although you might expect to have to avoid this type of restaurant altogether for the duration of the programme, you don't. Steak houses offer a large variety of foods that fit very nicely into the Good Mood Diet. Just be very careful about portion sizes. The protein part of your main course will almost always be at least two times larger than you should be eating.

Lunch, all phases: Grilled fish; grilled lean beef; steamed vegetables such as broccoli or asparagus; large mixed salad.

Dinner, phase 1: Baked potato with 1 teaspoon butter or 2 teaspoons soured cream and steamed vegetables; large mixed, spinach or chopped salad (no blue cheese, bacon or Caesar dressings) and bread.

Dinner, phases 2 and 3: Same as phase 1 plus an appetizer of grilled scallops, prawn cocktail or oysters on the half shell. Or eat part of a small beef fillet and carry home the rest for the next day's lunch.

Avoid: Creamed vegetables, béarnaise sauce, beurre blanc sauce, mashed potatoes and crab cakes.

Fast-Food Chains

At times, even the most dedicated avoider of fast-food chains may find that they are the only alternative to fasting for the next 8 hours. By following these suggestions, you will be able to stay close to the parameters of the diet, depending on the type of fast-food chain you go to.

Lunch, all phases: Any salad with deli meat; grilled chicken (as long as it's not 'crispy' or breaded); beef; skimmed milk; fruit.

Dinner, phase 1: Mixed green salad (don't eat the taco shell if it comes with one); vegetarian wrap sandwich without mayonnaise, cheese or sauce; vegetarian sandwich without cheese; baked potato with 1 teaspoon butter or 2 teaspoons soured cream and chives and vegetables or salad if available; vegetable pizza with cheese scraped off (do not order stuffed crust); kid-size ice cream cone.

Dinner, phases 2 and 3: Salad with dressing on the side; grilled chicken or lean beef on a roll with lettuce and tomato (no cheese); turkey sub with lettuce, tomato and green pepper (no mayo or cheese).

Avoid: Fried items such as french fries, chicken nuggets and fish sandwiches; cheese; soured cream; guacamole; stuffed-crust pizza; and cream-based soups.

NOW WHAT DO YOU DO?

Sometimes your usual routine will be disrupted, resulting in the foods you should eat not being available or the timing of meals being thrown off by travel, work, family, social events or other time pressures. Many situations will make you wonder how you're supposed to be able to follow the Good Mood Diet.

There will always be unexpected or even predictable situations that present obstacles to sticking to the diet's guidelines. With that in mind, here are a number of familiar 'Now what do I do?' scenarios. We give you solutions for all of them.

The No-Dinner Flight

The age of in-flight dining is over. Now what do you do?

1. Buy an oversized sandwich and a cinnamon bun with extra butter at the airport and wolf them down before the flight.

2. Wait until you check into your hotel and then, starving, order a pepperoni pizza with creamy coleslaw from room service.

3. If you are allowed to carry drinks and food on the plane, pick up a vegetarian wrap and fresh orange juice from one of the airport terminal cafes to take with you. When you get to the hotel, if you feel that you need more carbohydrate, eat the snack you packed.

The answer is number 3. Look for foods in the airport food court or departure terminal that contain some carbohydrate and vegetables. Options vary with the size of the airport. They may include vegetarian sushi, rice and vegetables, spaghetti with tomato sauce and salad, pizza with mushrooms and broccoli (try to scrape off most of the cheese), tomato or vegetable soup, salad and fresh bread, and tomato and mozzarella sandwiches on thick rolls. None of these options is perfect, but any one of them will eliminate your hunger without forfeiting your adherence to the diet.

Packing extra snacks is important because you may not be able to get all the carbohydrate you need from an airport meal, which will leave you full but not satisfied. Crunchy cereal bars are good choices because they are packable, have an extremely long shelf life, and are satisfying. If you forget them, you usually can buy them at a newspaper concession in the airport (although they will cost twice as much there as they do in your local supermarket).

The Wedding Reception

It is 4:30 p.m., 2 hours after the ceremony. No food, with the exception of a few high-calorie canapés, has been served – and those are long gone. You have just been seated for dinner, but there is nothing on the table except flowers. Since you're not sure whether they are edible, you leave them alone. Now what do you do?

1. Duck out and race to the bar, where you buy two packets of peanuts. Wolf them down before going back to your table.

2. Find a waitress and state that you must eat something because your metabolic condition requires food on schedule (just don't mention that the condition is called hunger). Ask if rolls and the first course could be served.

3. Grab the snack in your pocket or handbag, say you must make a phone call, and go someplace private to eat your food.

The answer is number 2 or 3, or both. When you are going to an event where the food may not appear for hours, be prepared. Not only should you eat your snack before leaving home – even if it is not the most appropriate time to do so – you should also carry a snack with you.

If you think the meal will be very late, have a small meal, like a bowl of cereal and a fruit, before going out so you will not be ravenous.

And don't forget the option of speaking up and asking that food be brought to your table. Diabetics do this all the time if their insulin treatments are tied to a particular meal schedule. Everyone else at the table will thank you.

No Time for a Workout

Your meeting went into overtime and you have only 45 minutes for your workout. Now what do you do?

1. Sacrifice the gym and visit the vending machine so you can vent your frustration by eating sweets.

2. Blow off steam by commiserating with your colleagues and hope you can wake up early enough the next morning to get to the gym before work.

3. Put on your walking shoes and do a 30-minute power walk followed by 10 minutes of exercises in your office with the door closed. Do lunges, press-ups, sit-ups and yoga stretches, all of which will help to energize you for the rest of the day.

The answer is, of course, number 3 because even a short workout is better than none at all. If the weather is too hot or cold to go outside, walk the halls of your building or, if they are accessible, climb the stairs. Doing the latter gives you a great workout in a short time. If exercising leaves you with no time to eat, have your lunch or a protein bar or shake at your desk.

Family Obligations

Your not-at-all-athletic in-laws are visiting and they intend to spend every minute with you and your kids. You are concerned that you will have to skip your weekend workouts. Now what do you do?

1. Tell your spouse that you'll be missing in action for 1 hour each weekend day so you can exercise.

2. Skip your workouts because your in-laws are coming from far away and you would feel guilty for taking so much time for yourself.

3. Plan a fun event for your family and in-laws to do while you exercise.

You can do number 1 or number 3 depending on your spouse's relationship with his or her parents. You may have to compromise and exercise for a shorter period of time or give up the idea of doing so every day. However, your mental and physical states will be enhanced if you continue to work out on a regular basis.

The 'We'll Eat at the Meeting' Lunch

The business meeting unexpectedly goes through lunch and a secretary comes in to take pizza orders. Now what do you do?

1. Order what everyone else is getting and then grab the biggest slice, followed by a second.

2. Ask the secretary to get you a large salad from the same place. Skip the pizza altogether.

3. Excuse yourself and go back to your desk for either the lunch you brought or your trusty protein bar and apple. Then rejoin everyone and eat your choice along with a bottle of water. If you opt for the protein bar and apple, have a pot of yogurt after the meeting.

Either number 2 or number 3 would be an appropriate choice. If you mention that you would rather have a salad – if possible with some grilled chicken or salmon – instead of the pizza, you will likely find that others at the meeting will ask for the same thing. If you don't want to disrupt the meeting by stipulating your dietary needs, excuse yourself, go to the person ordering the food, and ask that a salad be brought in for you.

Conventions, Exhibitions, Conferences

Your business travels take you to places where the featured foods are bathed in grease. Convention centres are rarely near a supermarket. Now what do you do?

1. Admit defeat and order fried onion rings and a huge hot dog at the food concession in the conference hall.
2. Starve yourself all day, figuring you'll be able to eat correctly at night. Then blow your diet once you begin eating.
3. Ask the hotel to prepare a packed lunch for you.
4. Walk around the exhibition hall and help yourself to the free goodies that exhibitors give away at their booths.

The answer is number 3. Meetings pose major food-selection problems for exhibitors and attendees. Often there is not enough time to order and eat a meal in a nearby restaurant because there are always too few dining venues for the number of people who want to eat lunch at the same time.

If you are staying at a hotel with room service, order a sandwich that can be eaten cold and ask that it be packed for you to take with you. You can travel with lunchbox-size ice packs that will fit in a small bag and keep your meal fresh at the exhibition hall. Or, when you pack for your trip, in addition to all the materials you'll need for the meeting or exhibit, add some protein bars and bananas, carrots, apples and low-fat snacks.

Many people contend that it is too much of a bother to do this. However, when you think about the planning and expense that goes into exhibiting or giving a paper, then spending a little time and money on a healthy lunch seems like a bargain.

End-of-the-Week Drinks

After a long, tough week, you and your friends look forward to Friday night. Before you were on a diet, you would consume your supper calories in the form of wine or cocktails and bar snacks. Now that you are on the Good Mood Diet, you are not sure that you will enjoy yourself unless you continue to eat and drink without regard for calories. Now what do you do?

1. Decide to skip dinner and have your calories in the form of creamy liqueur drinks and peanuts.
2. Munch on pretzels and drink soda water, feeling miserable and hungry and not at all like partying.
3. Eat before you go out so you can ignore the food and nurse a glass of white wine all evening.
4. Order a white wine spritzer and share a low-fat high-carb snack with a friend.

The answer is 3 or 4. Even though diets should not restrict you from participating in your normal social activities and it can be a challenge to 'party' and control calories, it is not impossible. One (or even two) wine spritzer is low in calories.

It's a good idea to eat something before going out so you won't be tempted to munch on the high-calorie offerings. Plus, you will be able to focus solely on the socializing. If your meal comes from the bar, try to order something that is relatively low in fat. Potato skins are not ideal because they are usually fried, but they are preferable to fried chicken wings. If the bar has a restaurant, ask the bartender to bring you a full menu so you can order a salad or another low-fat item.

The Celebratory Dinner

For your birthday, you are being taken to a restaurant known for its large portions. You feel you should order whatever you want since it is a celebration. But you know you will overeat. What really worries you is the bread basket, which is filled with delicious varieties of rolls and breads. In the past you ate almost everything in the basket and you are afraid you will be tempted to do that now. Now what do you do?

1. Order an appetizer rather than the main course or split a main-course selection with someone. Then eat all the rolls you can because the size of your main course is small.

2. Make sure that you eat your snack ahead of time. Then order a main course, but eat only half and take the other half home.

3. Tell yourself that your birthday comes only once a year and eat everything, including a large piece of cheesecake for dessert.

4. Take home half of the main course and ask the waiter if you can also have the remaining bread in the basket (after checking with your companions to make sure they don't want any).

The best option is 4 because it will give you two meals from your dinner out, plus you will not go over your calorie limit. Bread is not supposed to be recycled to another table, so do not be embarrassed about taking it home. Have it with soup or a large salad the next day.

The Awards Dinner

You are invited to a catered awards dinner. The meal consists of a tossed green salad, a small steak, baby carrots, a layered cheese and potato dish, and a soft roll. Dessert is a small piece of very rich chocolate cake with raspberry sauce. Red and white wines are also served. Now what do you do?

1. Eat everything, including the dessert, and drink two glasses of wine because the portions look small and you can go back on the diet tomorrow.

2. Ask one of the servers to bring you a vegetarian option. Request fruit instead of the cake.

3. Eat the salad, the roll, the carrots and the potatoes and wish you had the nerve to ask for a carry-home bag for the steak. Drink the wine because it is a type of carbohydrate.

4. Pour a tiny bit of dressing on the salad before you eat it along with the roll and half of the steak, all the carrots, and the part of the potato dish that is not soaked in melted cheese and

butter. Tell the waiter not to give you the cake so you will not be tempted by it. Sip at the wine, but consume only half a glass. When you get home, because you have been so attentive to the diet and because you want to relax from the festivities, allow yourself some Skinny Cow ice cream.

Option 2, 3 or 4 works, with some being better than others. Many people ask for special meals for medical (such as an allergy) or religious reasons. Often when beef is served, a vegetarian option is available since many people do not eat red meat. Plus, even a busy kitchen can plate some vegetables with potatoes or rice and serve you a dinner-size salad. The cake and wine are the only two elements of the meal that should be treated with caution, because they are totally empty calories. However, if you eat small amounts of everything that is served – except the cake – your diet will not suffer.

Note that boredom during after-dinner speeches causes people to pick at their dessert even if they had not planned on eating it. If dessert is not in front of you, you will not start eating it after the fourth long-winded address.

A Meltdown Is Imminent

Frustration over financial pressures, family strains or a work situation is pushing you to your limit. You want to eat everything in sight. Now what do you do?

1. Down a tub of ice cream, a big bar of chocolate or a super-size bag of crisps because it seems to be the only solution.
2. Have a snack even if it is not your traditional snack time. Then choose one – and only one – nonfood activity to distract you until the urge to overeat passes.
3. Give up on the diet because life is too stressful.

Option 2 is the answer. A snack will give you a serotonin boost, but it will take at least 10 minutes for it to kick in. In the meantime, you need something to distract you. Make sure whatever it is that you do is away from the kitchen or other sources of food.

For instance, sit down and write a 'to do' list, take out a sketch pad and some charcoal and draw, or reapply your nail polish.

The object is to take your mind off the immediate hassle and your automatic response to eat. If you still want to eat after the snack and 10 minutes of distraction, have another snack. Subtract the calories from the next meal, even if it is breakfast.

You can be on the diet and lose weight no matter how stressful life seems. The key is to eat to reduce your stress even if it means just maintaining your weight rather than losing weight.

FREQUENTLY ASKED QUESTIONS

I don't get home from the gym until 8 p.m. at the earliest. Am I supposed to eat dinner and a snack if I'm in phase 1 of the diet?

Yes. You should have your snack before going to the gym and plan on eating something that can be made quickly when you get home. If your gym has a snack bar that serves healthy vegetable salads along with grain salads and bread, eat before you go home. Otherwise, plan on eating something that can be made quickly, like soup, bread and a salad or a baked potato. You can freeze cooked rice or pasta and microwave it. Even a few slices of toast with jam, some tomato and cucumber slices, and a piece of fruit will be sufficient if you are tired and don't want to cook. But the best thing is to plan ahead and have food ready to eat when you arrive home. If you are in phase 1 of the programme, enjoy your after-dinner snack an hour or so before bedtime. If you don't finish dinner until just before you go to sleep, you can skip that snack.

My family isn't on the diet with me and they give me grief about it. How can I keep their attitude from sabotaging my efforts?

It isn't easy to remain on a diet when those around you do not support your efforts or even try to stop you from losing weight. You should speak to each family member privately to explain how important losing weight is for your health. Find out why there is such resistance to your dieting efforts. It may be because when you were on diets in the past you asked your family to give up foods they liked so that such temptations wouldn't be in the house. Reassure each family member that only your food choices are going to change; they can continue eating as usual. If you force them to follow your diet plan, say, for example, by eating only carbs and vegetables for dinner, they will resent it. So prepare meals that give them the foods they want, but make sure the meals contain the carbohydrate and low-fat protein you should be eating. Once your weight loss becomes obvious, everyone likely will be happy for you. Remember the saying 'Success has many fathers, but failure is an orphan.'

I'm very close to my aunt, who cooks a huge family Sunday dinner consisting of meat, a cheesy potato dish, carrots glazed with lots of butter and sugar, and cake for dessert. What can I eat without hurting her feelings?

If the meal is served in the afternoon, treat it as lunch; if it is served in the evening, treat it as dinner.

Before arriving, call your aunt and explain that you are trying to lose weight and must avoid eating certain foods for now. Ask if you can bring some dishes that fit into the diet plan to share with everyone. For instance, a large salad or a variety of roasted vegetables would be appropriate so you'll have something to eat along with the meat. If you can, take some pasta or rice salad or bread to share so you will not be tempted to eat the cheese and potato dish.

The cake will be tempting, but explain that you are trying to avoid sugar and extra fat. If she is upset that you are not partaking, tell her that you will take a couple of slices and enjoy them during the week after a lighter meal. Bring the slices to work the next day and give them to your colleagues. Or just throw them away.

Finally, you can attempt to control the entire meal situation by telling your aunt that you would like to reciprocate for all of her hospitality. Offer to take her out at least one Sunday a month. That way you will be able to follow the diet without preplanning, and you'll give her a break, too.

I've been following the diet, but I face the same situation every day. I snack an hour before lunch, which usually consists of turkey on a slice of bread and a huge salad with 2 teaspoons of light dressing. But around 45 minutes later I get so stressed – there is a daily afternoon meeting that is very stressful. When I walk out of the meeting I want to eat again. Do I eat more carbs although it's not snack time?

IT'S EASIER THAN YOU MAY THINK
TO MAKE THE RIGHT CHOICES

To give you an idea of how many calories you save by eating lean, look at the calorie comparisons of these foods.

Subway Spicy Italian sandwich: **491 calories**

Subway Veggie Delite sandwich: **210 calories**

Cheese pizza, thin crust, 2 slices: **280 calories**

Cheese pizza, thin crust, 2 slices blotted to absorb excess oil: **235 calories**

McDonald's Double Cheeseburger:**445 calories**

McDonald's Chicken Ranch Salad: **250 calories**

Mayonnaise, 1 tablespoon: **100 calories**

Light mayonnaise, 1 tablespoon: **50 calories**

Salami, 30 g (1 oz): **105 calories**

Lean ham, 30 g (1 oz): **37 calories**

Tuna, chunk light in oil, 90 g (3 oz): **165 calories**

Tuna, chunk light in water, 90 g (3 oz): **90 calories**

Latte with whole milk, 240 ml (8 fl oz): **130 calories**

Latte with skimmed milk, 240 ml (8 fl oz): **80 calories**

Greek-style natural yogurt with honey (140 g pot): **205 calories**

Fat-free natural yogurt (150 g pot), with 75 g (2½ oz) blueberries: **129 calories**

Streaky bacon, 1 rasher (20 g) grilled: **74 calories**

Back bacon, 1 rasher (28 g) grilled: **49 calories**

Spare ribs, 90 g (3 oz): **315 calories**

Pork chop, 90 g (3 oz): **172 calories**

There are a couple of ways to solve this problem. If your most stressful time is midafternoon, you could eat only carbs and vegetables at lunch during the week. You would eat your dinner portion of carbohydrate at lunchtime and follow the lunch options for dinner. (A client who was a teacher did this because her stress and its accompanying overeating occurred during the school day rather than when she got home at night.) If you decide to do this, then eat your snack right after the meeting instead of eating it before lunch. Then eat your second snack about an hour before dinner.

The other option is to eat the snack about an hour before the meeting begins so you will be calm when you go into it. Then lunch can follow the meeting.

Along with these two possibilities, you can subdue your anxiety after the meeting with 2 minutes of meditation or relaxation in your office or by leaving the building for a brisk walk.

I must eat chocolate every day. A bar of chocolate or a slice of chocolate cake is the highlight of my day. Why can't I eat chocolate on this diet?

The problem with using chocolate as a serotonin-boosting snack is its high fat content, which will delay the digestion of its carbohydrate content and your brain's production of more serotonin. However, many of the snack options on the diet are chocolate-flavoured. There are lots of ways to obtain the flavour you seek without the added fat and calories. But if you want to occasionally treat yourself to a small amount of chocolate, you can, especially if you have exercised off a lot of calories. But pick the chocolate carefully. Make sure it is a small portion and that you eat only one serving.

I am fine on the diet until right before I get my period. Then I go crazy for chocolate. What can I do?

You are probably suffering from premenstrual carbohydrate cravings; it is known that serotonin is involved in these feelings. Follow the Serotonin Surge diet during that time. If you must have chocolate, drink some fat-free hot chocolate or experiment with a chocolate-flavoured breakfast cereal.

PART THREE

PLANNING

YOUR STRATEGY

CHAPTER NINE

The 12-Week Guide

O ur guide is a road map for the trip to successful weight loss. It will serve as a map, a set of directions and a global positioning system (GPS) to show you where you are at all times, even when you feel like you are lost.

We know where you should be during this 12-week process, so we can advise you on when your dieting should continue on the same path, change direction, or go off on an interesting side trip or to the service stop. You don't have to check in continually to find out where you are or where you should go next, but we think you should look at the guide at least once a week. You will track your weight loss, check where you are on the map, update your navigation and follow our road signs to help you stay on course, even if you've been unable to follow the diet perfectly.

GETTING STARTED: WEEK 1

Just as with any road journey, you have to prepare before you start. Buy a notebook to help you work through the 12-week guide. Any notebook will do.

The first thing you must do is weigh yourself. Do this either the day before or the day you start the diet. Weigh yourself in the morning before breakfast. Always wear the same thing: nothing, a towel, or your underwear.

Record the date and your weight. You will be doing this on the same day of each week until the end of the diet.

Your notebook might look like this:

Date: January 15

Weight: 82 kg

Weight lost: _____ [You will fill this in each week starting with week 2.]

Read over the diet guidelines for phase 1, Serotonin Surge, starting on page 74. It is useful to photocopy or write down the basic guidelines and keep them in your notebook. Beginning the Good Mood Diet without them is like starting on your journey without your map.

Use the sample menus and snack lists to figure out what you will be eating for each meal. If you eat away from home, decide what you can order that will fit within the diet guidelines.

Go food shopping for the meal and snack foods you will be eating.

Pack snacks to take with you if snack time will occur when you are away from home.

Leave your measuring scales out on the worktop so it is easy to measure what you are eating. Buy a set of scales if you don't have them; it is very important to know how much you are eating.

Remove or hide all tempting foods in the house, car and your desk drawers at work. (Do not remove them by eating them!)

You are on your way.

Road Signs

1. Every morning, take 5 minutes or so to review what you will be eating for meals and snacks that day.

2. Don't leave the house without your snacks and lunch if you eat them away from home.

3. Be sure to measure your food at meals as often as you can (we don't expect you to weigh food in a restaurant). If you don't know how much you are eating, you may end up eating less than you should. This is especially true of the dinner carbohydrates.

Road Assistance

1. Strategically place reminders to have your snacks on time.

2. Don't forget to eat breakfast, even if you are not used to eating

in the morning. Take it with you if you are in too much of a rush to eat it before leaving home.

3. Be proud of yourself for being on the Good Mood Diet. It is challenging, and you should feel good about starting this journey and doing something positive for yourself.

Road Blocks

Are you hoping that just wanting to lose weight will be enough to make it happen? If you don't change the way you eat, you won't change your waistline.

WEEK 2

Weigh yourself and write the date, your weight and the amount of weight you've lost in your notebook.

You've made it through the first week and are getting used to the landscape. Congratulations. You may have lost some weight, but it's also possible that you didn't lose any weight during this first week. Don't worry, and do not use this as a reason to abandon the Good Mood Diet! It takes time for your body to efficiently use stored body fat, which is what translates into real weight loss. Stick with the plan and you will soon be losing 0.5–1 kg (1–2 lb) or more per week.

Road Signs

1. Review the sample menus and recipes. Many of our clients enjoy the diversity of the recipes and find them extremely satisfying.

2. Review the exercise guidelines in Chapter 7.

3. Check the condition of your walking or running shoes. If they are worn at the heel or the cushioning is gone, buy another pair. Old shoes can cause new aches and pains.

4. Spend 10 minutes a day doing some sort of physical activity. Walking is a good start. Do more if you have the time and energy.

Road Assistance

1. Check your snack supplies to make sure others in the house have not demolished them.

2. Resist the temptation to eat protein at dinner; save it for lunch. It will taste just as good.

3. Feel too tired to exercise in the afternoon? Have your snack, wait 20 minutes and then walk. You will feel a burst of serotonin-charged energy. Take a walk at lunch, or wake up 10 minutes earlier and walk in the morning.

4. Tired of drinking plain water? Try fruit-flavoured zero-calorie water drinks.

5. Activate and use your support system. Family members, friends, neighbours and colleagues can help you stay on track and be there to share your successes.

6. Congratulate yourself – you made it through another week.

Road Blocks

1. Are you forgetting to do your daily planning for meals and snacks? If you keep snacks along with protein bars, tuna in a pouch, crackers and dry cereal in your drawer or locker at work and carrots, yogurt, cottage cheese and juice in the company refrigerator, you will prevent yourself from going to the vending machine or nearest shop for breakfast, lunch and snacks when your day is really frantic.

2. No time for a walk? Block off some time on your calendar. Get off the bus one stop early and walk the rest of the way. Walk to do your errands or park far from your destination.

WEEK 3

Week 3 moves you into the second phase of the Good Mood Diet programme: the Serotonin Balance phase. Think of it as entering the motorway for the longest part of the journey.

Weigh yourself and write the date, your weight and the amount of weight you've lost in your notebook.

Road Signs

1. Review the Serotonin Balance diet guidelines on page 82 to 83.

2. Note that you will be eating slightly less protein at lunch and adding a small amount of protein to dinner.

3. Use the sample menus to decide what to eat for lunch and dinner. Be sure to measure the protein, because it is very easy to underestimate how much you are eating.

4. Eliminate the evening snack, but continue to eat the late-morning and late-afternoon snacks on schedule.

5. Pay attention to when you want to snack in the afternoon. Eat the snack as soon as you notice your cravings coming on so they don't overwhelm you. That way, you will not have to use willpower to prevent yourself from eating snacks not on the Good Mood Diet.

6. Increase your exercise time. Walk briskly or do some other energetic physical activity for 20 to 30 minutes each day. This can be cleaning the house, climbing stairs or doing some exercises while watching the nightly news. If you do not have time to do it all at once, break it up into 10-minute segments.

Road Assistance

1. Buy a pedometer to track your walking. Keep it on every day, including weekends. Aim for 10,000 steps a day (this translates into approximately 5 miles that you can rack up throughout the day without ever setting foot on a treadmill). You can build up to this goal gradually. You'll feel better about yourself, and the extra calories burned will translate into speedier weight loss.

2. Keep a pair of walking shoes at work so you can take a quick 20-minute walk at lunchtime.

3. When shopping, take your snacks with you. Otherwise, the temptation of all those coffee shops and sandwich bars in the high street or shopping centre may be too great.

4. If you can't watch TV or movies at home without eating, take up a hobby that keeps both hands busy, like knitting, crocheting or other craft work.

Road Blocks

1. If you used to spend your evenings nibbling or fighting with yourself about eating, you may be forgetting to do things that make you feel good about yourself. Identify some way to relax and reward yourself, particularly if your day has been stressful or overly busy.

2. Prevent yourself from eating leftovers by immediately putting the food in containers in the fridge or freezer after you serve your meal. If food still tempts you after your meal, do something for at least a half hour: read the newspaper, check your e-mail, phone a friend.

3. Too much to do and too little time to do it? Don't eat while you decide what to do next. Prioritize and pick one thing to focus on. Then forget about the rest for the time being. It can wait until you're done with the task at hand.

WEEK 4

Weigh yourself and write the date, your weight and the amount of weight you've lost in your notebook.

Road Signs

1. When you are driving on a long stretch of road with little traffic, it is easy to go considerably above the speed limit, especially if everyone else is doing so. It is just as easy to eat too-large portion sizes, especially in restaurants, because everyone else is doing so. Few restaurants today serve food in quantities that will satisfy nutritional needs without giving you excess calories.

2. You have to train yourself to estimate serving sizes. When you eat at home, measure what you serve yourself so you'll know what a portion of the correct size looks like. This skill comes in handy when you are eating at someone else's home, especially if it's a relative who likes to serve huge portions.

3. Read food labels. Look at serving size, calories, and protein, fat, and carbohydrate contents. You may find that you are not eating enough (a happy thought) or that a snack or prepared food that

you thought was low in calories is low-calorie only when you eat a small sliver.

4. Check restaurant food ingredients. Chapter 8 gives you ideas for what to order, but you must check for yourself. You can consume more calories than you intended to due to hidden fat ingredients in restaurant food.

5. For physical activity to be most effective for weight loss, you should now increase its intensity (unless you are limited by a physical condition). During one exercise session this week, push yourself in an aerobic activity for at least 30 minutes continuously.

6. Add muscle to your exercise programme. Now is the time to add strength training. If you are already doing so, that's terrific. Keep it up. Otherwise, keep up your 20 to 30 minutes of exercise a day and add 30 minutes of strength training, either in one session or broken into shorter sessions throughout the week.

Road Assistance

1. Join a gym or health club that offers a free fitness evaluation and training on equipment.

2. Never hesitate to ask a trainer how to use a piece of equipment.

3. Do yoga as a first step toward muscle strengthening. Your arms and back will show results very quickly.

4. Take a few minutes to read the recipes for lunch and dinner. Dieting *can* taste good – particularly if you use the Good Mood Diet recipes.

5. Have you done something nice for yourself this week? You should. You have reached the 4-week point. Congratulations! Go to the cinema with a friend, or take time to relax without thinking about your to-do list.

Road Blocks

1. Unexpected weight gain? Are you eating foods with a lot of salt? Do you have PMS this week? Check pages 155 to 163 in the troubleshooting chapter to see what might be the problem.

2. Spending late afternoons at home can be a prescription for over-eating. If your nibbling wants to go up as the sun goes down, get out of the kitchen. This is a good time to exercise. Your body will feel more energetic and your mood will improve.

3. Long winter evenings are also an inducement for many people to overeat. Now is the time to sign up for activities that will lessen the amount of time you spend at home. Check your newspaper for weekly events.

4. Feeling frustrated because you expected to lose more weight by now? Remember that you are losing fat, not water. A 0.5–1 kg (1–2 lb) weight loss each week is right on target.

WEEK 5

Weigh yourself and write the date, your weight and the amount of weight you've lost in your notebook.

Road Signs

1. Experiment with new foods and recipes to alleviate boredom. Colour your diet with vegetables. In general, the more colourful the vegetable, the more nutrients it contains. Try beetroot, kale, watercress, cabbage, red peppers, broccoli, sweet potatoes, green beans, artichokes, aubergine, asparagus, spinach, peas and mangetout.

2. Use recipe books, magazines and food sites on the Web to learn how to prepare vegetables that are unfamiliar. Ask friends for cooking tips, or ask a restaurant's chef how he or she prepared a particularly good-tasting vegetable.

3. If social get-togethers leave you hungry because there is nothing to eat, bring Good Mood Diet-appropriate dishes. Many of the dinner recipes can be made in large quantities and will appeal to everyone's tastes.

4. Increase the intensity of your muscle-strengthening exercise so your muscles feel tired. Aim for 1 hour of strength training over the course of the week. A fatigued muscle today is a stronger muscle tomorrow.

5. In addition to walking as much as possible every day, increase the intensity of your aerobic activity for at least 1 hour this week, either in one session or broken down into shorter sessions throughout the week.

Road Assistance

1. Exercise must be convenient; otherwise, you will find reasons not to do it. Would you brush your teeth as much as you do if you had to drive 10 miles to use a toothbrush?

2. Create a back-up exercise plan if you know that time, obligations, weather or travel may interfere with daily physical activity. An exercise DVD is a good substitute for a brisk walk when your babysitter lets you down. A treadmill indoors beats running outdoors when it's baking hot. Resistance bands can be tucked into the corner of your suitcase so you can do some toning exercises in your hotel room while watching the news. At the playground with the kids? Pushing your toddler on the swing is a good arm movement. Run races with your kids or exercise with your dog. All of you will benefit. (See Chapter 7 for more tips.)

3. Increase your exercise gradually to avoid injury and remember that it takes time to see significant weight loss and body-shape changes.

4. Consider weighing yourself daily as a reminder to stay on track. But don't do daily weigh-ins if the number on the scale might trigger overeating.

Road Blocks

1. Spending your disposable time on planning your meals and snacks and exercising may seem like a big sacrifice, especially once the novelty of being on the diet has passed. But, as with any new habit, the more you do it, the faster and more efficient you become. Stick with the new eating and exercise routines; soon your new lifestyle will seem easy and natural.

2. If you get bored while you exercise, try multi-tasking. Return phone calls on your mobile while walking. At home, listen to

books on tape, watch the news or catch up on the latest sitcom while using an exercise bike. A client of ours used to rent DVDs of movies she was otherwise too busy to see.

3. Plan activities for the times in your week when you need to refresh yourself mentally and emotionally. Take time to relax and distract yourself with pleasurable activities. Paying bills or calling your relatives doesn't count.

WEEK 6

Weigh yourself and write the date, your weight and the amount of weight you've lost in your notebook.

Road Signs

1. What rewards are you giving yourself each week for successfully staying on the diet and exercising? If you have not identified any substitutes that are as good as or better than the meal or snack that used to be your reward, start immediately to give yourself some. As you think of small favours you can do for yourself instead of eating, you will realize that these pleasures last much longer than the taste of a meal or snack.

2. Dieting is about making the right choices. And that means deciding to forgo certain things you might otherwise enjoy if you weren't on the Good Mood Diet. You cannot eat everything you want and you cannot skip exercising. Tough choices like these allow you to reap some very sweet rewards, like being slimmer and having a more fit physique.

3. To get you through the more challenging times, spend time with people you care about and who care about you. This is also a good time to think about other positive changes you can make. Why not go to the library and explore your options. You may decide you want a new career; take the courses needed to make this a reality. Alternatively, you may find you simply become engrossed in a good book. The goal is to find something that adds pleasure, joy and meaning to your day, week and month.

4. This week, increase the amount of more intense aerobic activity to 90 minutes, ideally divided into three 30-minute sessions.

5. Increase the amount of strength training you do to 90 minutes spread out over the course of the week. For example, you can go to a 1-hour body-toning class at the gym and spend 10 minutes on 3 other days doing hand-weight exercises, such as lunges and biceps curls, at home.

Road Assistance

1. Exercise is even more important at this point in the diet. You must continue to increase both the duration and intensity of your strength training. Dieting always results in some muscle loss, and if you do not build it back up with exercise, your metabolism may slow down and your body will not look its toned and shapely best.

2. Measuring what you are eating is also extremely important during the second half of the diet programme. You can be sure that your weight will reflect every meal or snack you have overeaten.

3. Don't let people tell you that your face has gotten so thin that you should stop the diet. They are probably jealous that they have not been able to lose weight as successfully as you have.

4. Change snacks if you have been eating the same foods for the past several weeks. And make sure you continue to have two snacks a day.

5. Give yourself the present of a mental mini-break during a busy or stressful day. It will take no more than 2 minutes to restore your mental and emotional energy. Sit in a comfortable spot, place your hands flat on your chest and take two normal breaths. Then inhale deeply into your lungs as you count to four and slowly exhale as you again count to four. Repeat the cycle. Then move your hands to your belly and repeat the cycle twice. Remember, all it takes is 2 minutes for you to feel calm, contented and ready to face the next obligation. (This is also good when you're stuck in traffic.)

Road Blocks

1. Are there times when you consistently have trouble staying on the diet? Read through Chapter 10 for tips on removing common obstacles to following the diet guidelines.

2. Do a food search of your house, car and office. Have any high-calorie goodies been snuck in when you were not looking? Remove all temptations. If these foods have to stay in the house, make sure they are not visible. Out of sight, out of mouth.

3. Are you becoming bored with your exercising? Review Chapter 7 for suggestions on recreational activities that burn calories. You may have denied yourself the fun of physical activity before you started to lose weight because it was so tiring and maybe even painful. Now that you are fitter and stronger, you can go on a walking trip, climb the stairs to a monument or do some kayaking. Owners of MP3 players can vary their routines by downloading personal fitness and training programmes from the Web.

4. Are you still doing your daily planning for meals and snacks? What about planning your exercise? Do you need to pack your gym clothes in advance, call a friend to schedule a power walk, or schedule a spinning class at the gym? Without a plan, you may falter, especially those of you who would rather get a tooth pulled than get on a treadmill.

WEEK 7

Congratulations! You are entering the second half of the weight-loss trip. It is important at this point to make sure there are no U-turns in your adherence to the diet. There must be no turning back to gaining weight, to overeating behaviour, or to making excuses for not exercising. You will be on this journey to the end and we will be with you for every mile.

Weigh yourself and write the date, your weight and the amount of weight you've lost in your notebook.

Road Signs

1. Long trips inevitably prompt the question 'Are we there yet?' When it is apparent that the destination is not yet in sight, it is

hard to contain your impatience. Reaching your weight-loss goal can be just like that. No matter how motivated you were at the start, the journey may seem awfully long at this point. It is very tempting to turn off at the nearest exit and end the programme prematurely, or to decide to take a side trip to a quick weight-loss diet so you'll feel like you are reaching your goal sooner. Do neither.

2. Kids play games (or watch DVDs) during long trips. You should do stimulating and pleasurable activities so you'll associate this weight-loss interval with a productive and happy time. (One client made a quilt while she was losing weight; each square represented a 1-kg (2-lb) weight loss. Another started an elaborate garden at the beginning of the diet. Her joy at seeing her plants flower made the months of losing weight go by very quickly.)

3. In addition to continuing to move around as much as possible during the day, increase the time you spend on challenging exercise. This week, do a total of 2 hours of high-intensity aerobic exercise, physical limitations permitting, and keep up the 90 minutes of strength training you started last week. This is the level of exercise you will maintain throughout the rest of the Good Mood Diet.

Road Assistance

1. Take time to really taste your food, noticing its appearance, texture, temperature and smell. Remember how wonderful the first strawberry of the season tastes? Or the crunchy bite of a newly picked apple? Food should be enjoyed.

2. Have the seasons changed while you have been on the diet? Make a seasonal adjustment of your menus and meal planning. Switch to vegetable-packed soups rather than salads if it is cold outside, or grill red peppers and sweetcorn on a warm summer night.

3. Bank holidays and occasions like birthdays, weddings or anniversaries may make you take a holiday from the diet. That is fine as long as you eat the non-Good Mood Diet food in moderation and go back on the diet tomorrow.

Road Blocks

1. Friends and family can be even more impatient than you are with your dieting. It would probably take another book to understand why comments like 'Are you still on your diet? You look too thin' or 'Eat this, it won't hurt you' are thrown at you rather than support and understanding. Pay no attention. You are the one who stands on the scales, not them. You are the one who is wearing smaller-size clothing, climbing stairs without panting and walking away from high-calorie temptations. So when these comments come, just smile (or grit your teeth) and change the subject.

2. If your dieting and exercise come up against the obstacles of work, family or social crises, don't give up; just do the best you can. It is like running into roadworks on the motorway; you will be slowed down and get to your destination a little later, but you will still get there.

3. Are you longing to taste some foods you have not had for almost 2 months? Go ahead. A small portion of whatever you are longing for will not affect your weight loss and it will make your taste buds happy for another few weeks. Caution: if you think you can't stop with a small portion, don't start.

4. Are you afraid that exercise will be harmful in some way, that you will strain your back lifting weights or damage your knees while jogging? The solution is to take on activities that you feel comfortable doing (if jogging is not your thing, don't do it) and to gradually increase the amount and intensity of your exercise. A professional or an experienced friend can show you what to do.

WEEK 8

Weigh yourself and write the date, your weight and the amount of weight you've lost in your notebook.

Road Signs

Sometimes focusing on overeating and your weight are ways of not thinking about the problems that caused the overeating. At this point in the diet, it is important to recognize the work, social or family situations that cause you to reach for food. You may have done so already. As was pointed out in Chapter 3, sometimes you can anticipate those situations that cause you to overeat and prevent them from occurring or minimize their impact.

However, problems that cannot be solved or negotiated away may trigger overeating after the diet is finished – for instance, a boss from hell, a horrible commute or an ageing parent with a chronic disability. The way to deal with such triggers is to recognize them for what they are. By identifying them, you can prevent them from destroying your control over eating.

An unexpected call from the nursing home administrator or an unjust criticism from the boss may make you reach automatically for food. Recognize what is happening. If you feel out of control, it is all right to eat a diet-appropriate carbohydrate snack. You may need more serotonin at this moment. In a few minutes you will feel calmer. Do not continue to eat. Eating more will not make the situation any better, nor will it improve your ability to deal with it. If you follow this advice, you will reach a healthier weight.

Road Assistance

1. Feel fidgety in the evening? Spend a few hours going through old photos and scrapbooks. Organize the photos on your computer into an album and add comments your kids will chuckle about in years to come.

2. Are weekends alone making it hard to stay on the diet? Many organizations – charity shops are a good example – are begging for volunteers on weekends. Many galleries and museums are free to the public. If you love movies, consider getting a part-time job at a local cinema. You'll get to watch all the movies for free, and get paid for doing it.

3. Go through your wardrobe and discard clothes that are now too big. Give them to a charitable organization. Do not leave them in your wardrobe 'in case' you gain weight.

4. If you find that you are hungry when you're food shopping, buy a snack (like a small roll) and eat it in the store. Just remember to pay for it.

5. If you're ravenous for a meal and it's only afternoon-snack time, consider having dinner at 4 p.m. and your afternoon snack at 7 p.m. One of our clients found this option to be an enormous relief and incredibly satisfying.

6. Get a heart-rate monitor to use while doing aerobic exercise. It will tell you when you're working hard enough to reach the fat-burning zone and give you something to focus on.

Road Blocks

1. Don't volunteer to do any baking for birthdays or other special occasions.

2. Appetizers offered at receptions are usually loaded with calories. Never depend on such food as a substitute for dinner. If the dinner that follows is going to be served late or not at all, consider eating at home before going.

3. Are you correctly portioning your snacks? Remember that endless handfuls of cereal or pretzels can lead to ingesting many unnecessary calories and no weight loss.

4. Are people annoying you with questions about how much weight you have lost and then telling you that someone they know lost more? Realize that they do not understand what you are going through or the importance of the changes you have made in your eating and exercise habits and in your self-knowledge. Just smile and change the subject.

5. Are you using your to-do list as an excuse not to focus on your eating and exercise? Take a look at your list of commitments to people, projects and daily tasks and decide what you are going to let go of. Even those of us who like to be in control of everything can indeed let go of something. Check your e-mail only twice a day. Delegate where possible: hire a cleaner so your weekends are not filled with endless housework, pay a neighbourhood teenager to mow the lawn, or talk to your boss if your workload is taking all of your free time. Plan your kids' schedules so you are not imprisoned in your car for 3 hours every afternoon. Say 'no' to activities you don't have time to do. Unless you're genuinely interested, don't volunteer to take on new work

or projects. Of course it's not always realistic to drop all burdensome obligations and commitments, but not striving to be superhuman can help your weight-loss efforts succeed.

WEEK 9

You are now going into the third and final phase of the diet plan, the Serotonin Control phase. This last part of the programme lasts 4 weeks, though it can be continued until you reach your weight-loss goal. This phase will help you make the transition into your post-diet, or maintenance, eating. The number of snacks is limited to one, but the good news is that you get to choose from a greater variety of foods. Eat the snack in the afternoon, as you have been doing all along. Chapter 5 provides guidance about the correct calorie and carbohydrate content of the snacks you should now be eating. You may switch to different snacks or continue to eat the same snacks as before, but now in smaller quantities.

Weigh yourself and write the date, your weight and the amount of weight you've lost in your notebook.

Road Signs

1. Enjoy experimenting with new snack foods, but be sure to adhere to the phase 3 calorie and carbohydrate content guidelines.

2. Trust your body to lose weight as long as you continue to follow the diet, exercise away your fat stores and rely on your brain to control your overeating. The only reasonable way of accelerating your weight loss is to significantly increase the duration and intensity of your exercise. For example, if you go on a week-long cycling trip, start training for long-distance races, or enter a ballroom dancing contest, you will lose more weight. If you don't have the time, talent or interest to do these activities, try adding a little more physical activity each day if you can.

3. During these next few weeks, take some time to think about the Road Blocks mentioned for earlier weeks and your success in resolving them. Make note of what or who has been most helpful and supportive of your weight loss. You should be extremely pleased with yourself; don't take any weight loss for granted.

It is challenging, and we applaud your achievements. Keep it up. Runners in a road race hear this encouragement all the time: 'You are almost there and looking good!'

Road Assistance

1. Are your workout clothes looking baggy? Maybe it is time to put on something a little sleeker. You deserve it.

2. Keep giving yourself rewards of free time and fun. Do something that makes you feel good, relaxed and happy every day. It can be as simple as sitting down and reading a magazine before you tackle the bills, giving yourself a pedicure or playing a card game with your kids. Wrestle with your dog or tease your cat with catnip. Just do something that may be a little silly and fun.

Road Blocks

1. You must keep measuring and weighing your food. Those portion sizes creep up, and if you are assuming that you are eating the same amount you ate weeks ago, you may be fooling yourself. The scales will know.

2. How is the exercise coming along? Have you increased the intensity? Does your pulse rate get high enough? Are you increasing the duration when you feel like doing more? Your body is fitter and stronger. Let the exercise reflect this.

3. Make sure you weigh yourself every week, even if you don't want to. See Chapter 10, on troubleshooting, if the scales are not moving downward. You are in the homestretch and we want to make sure you get to your goal.

WEEK 10

Weigh yourself and write the date, your weight and the amount of weight you've lost in your notebook.

Road Signs

You are almost at the end; don't abandon your journey now. You may be thinking that you have dieted for long enough, that you've lost some weight and don't want to be bothered with dieting and exercise for a while. It's understandable, but not a good idea. At this point in the programme, you are in control of your eating, you have formed an exercise habit, and you understand what triggers your overeating and what can prevent it. So why stop doing these activities that improve your health, give you more energy and make you calmer? Rejoice in your success and do something wonderful for yourself as a reward for coming this far on the journey to weight loss.

Road Assistance

1. Prevent yourself from eating too much at a social occasion by wearing something that just fits around your waist. If it is snug before dinner, you will resist making it snugger during dinner.

2. Boredom can push you into eating – even when you have no intention of doing so. Long flights, after-dinner speakers, reading work-related documents, studying for an exam, dull dining companions: the list of potential triggers is long. Taking frequent stretching breaks while doing tedious desk work or daydreaming your way through boring talks sometimes works. Rather than eating, just remember, 'This too shall pass'.

3. Change what you are doing for exercise. If you've been doing the same old thing, now is the time to try something new. Weather permitting, go outside to do the cycling, walking or running you have been doing in a gym or at home. Check out group recreational activities. Is there a cycling or walking group in your area? Are there weekend walking tours? Have you always wanted to learn how to canoe or mountain bike or belly dance? Sign up for a class at your gym or recreational centre. Stand in the back of the room if you feel shy.

Road Blocks

1. On days when everything goes wrong and all you want to do is eat chocolate or a bag of crisps, the Good Mood Diet may seem much less important than satisfying your need for the treats you used to eat when you were upset. If and when this happens, do this: eat one of the snacks from phase 1 and 2. You need the larger amount of carbohydrate right now. Then wait 20 minutes

without eating anything else. You should feel a little calmer. Do you still want the chocolate bar or crisps? If you do, then eat one small chocolate bar or a lunch-box-size bag of crisps and enjoy the taste and texture. Do not open a large bag of chocolate sweets or crisps. Leave areas where food is available and do something nice for yourself. The combination of the diet snack and the treat snack should make you feel more comfortable emotionally and will not damage your diet.

2. Has a cold or other illness sidetracked your exercise regime? When you start again, exercise at a more gentle level until you feel your strength returning. Your body may still be tired.

3. Sometimes weight loss slows down at this point in the diet as the body becomes accustomed to eating fewer calories. We know you will feel frustrated if this happens. But remember, you are still losing weight; it is just going to take a little longer to show up on the scales.

WEEK 11

Weigh yourself and write down the date, your weight and the amount of weight you've lost in your notebook.

Road Signs

Make an extra effort over these last 2 weeks to increase your weight loss before the programme ends. Think about what you will be eating to make sure that extra calories are not creeping into the meals or snacks. Exercise just a little harder so you work off more calories. Most people are thrilled when they lose a kilogram during the first weeks of a diet programme, but it is even more impressive to lose extra weight at the end. This is where exercise really matters. We have seen the results. And so have you.

Road Assistance

1. What are you eating for breakfast? Have you slipped back into eating only carbs and coffee? What happened to the protein? You will work more effectively during the morning if you give yourself time to eat our recommended breakfasts, and you won't

find yourself watching the clock to see if it is lunchtime.

2. Vegetable alert! We suspect you may not be eating all of your vegetables at this point. Lettuce really doesn't count for much. If you hate preparing vegetables, buy them already sliced or diced and frozen at your supermarket. Or get them from a salad bar or a café that specializes in good salads. All you need is a fork.

3. And now for protein. Are you eating too much of it at dinner? It is easy to slip back into making protein the main course. Don't. You need your carbohydrates. Your body may be thinner, but your brain still needs to make serotonin.

Road Blocks

1. Is the absence of a morning snack making you feel stressed and likely to nibble? Add it back into your diet plan. Your objective is to control your appetite and emotional overeating. Keep eating two snacks a day until you feel secure enough to drop the one in the morning.

2. Are you finding it difficult to control your snacking when you eat more interesting and tastier foods? Don't eat them as snacks. Return to the snacks you ate in the earlier phases of the diet plan. Many of us avoid certain foods all our lives because we know that if we start eating them, we will overeat them.

3. Do you have small children who interfere with your alone time? Buy them egg timers and set them for your own time-out. They will learn that 2 minutes is not forever.

WEEK 12

Weigh yourself and write the date, your weight and the amount of weight you've lost in your notebook.

Road Signs

The end of the programme is in sight. You are wonderful for sticking with the weight-loss plan and our advice for so long. End the week in style: wear your smaller-size clothes and show off your new physique. Follow the diet guidelines carefully so there are no slip-ups. And most importantly, think about how you have gained control over your appetite and your emotional overeating. If you are taking antidepressants, acknowledge how much control you now have over your eating. If you had been on a low-carbohydrate diet before starting this one, appreciate how easy it is to turn off your appetite without risk of eating large quantities of fatty foods.

You can continue with this phase of the diet for as long as you want to lose weight. When you reach your goal, you will enter the Maintenance phase.

Buy a full-length mirror. Admire your newly toned and energetic body. Keep it this way. Continue to schedule exercise into your calendar and aim to follow our weekly exercise prescription: at least 2 hours of challenging aerobic exercise and 90 minutes of strength training – only 3½ hours over the course of a week. And don't stop the moving around throughout the day that you've been doing, such as walking briskly rather than driving, and playing in the park with your kids. You have worked really hard to get to this point, and now you can enjoy the recreational activities that were difficult for you before you started on the weight-loss programme.

During this last week, give yourself and your brain credit for your weight loss, because you now know how to activate your appetite control with the foods you choose. You have learned how to handle stress by increasing serotonin. Your responsive brain subdues your anxiety and worries and allows you to let go of your concerns.

Enjoy yourself. Celebrate your achievement.

CHAPTER TEN

Troubleshooting

Life throws up unexpected events that can derail even the most determined Good Mood dieter. We know that you will face obstacles that will make it hard for you to stay committed every day. If you stumble, don't be discouraged. You are not alone. No one performs 'perfectly' every day – not Olympic champions, not movie stars, not even diet-book authors. Most importantly, when those events happen, do not judge yourself. You went off the rails a bit – but it doesn't mean you're a failure.

Diets, like cars and computers, do not always run smoothly. When that happens, there are simple ways to restart or reboot the Good Mood Diet to get it up and running again.

GETTING BACK ON TRACK

If you have not lost any weight, or if you've gained weight 2 weeks in a row, read this chapter to find out why that happened.

To help you pinpoint trouble spots during the week, keep a food diary for 3 weekdays and 1 weekend day. By writing down what you eat, you will see when you did not follow the diet guidelines by, for example, skipping or eating the wrong snacks or shirking on exercise.

Make sure that your food choices continue to be healthy. And continue, as much as possible, to eat the recommended carbohydrate snacks and carbohydrate dinners. Doing so will keep your brain serotonin level high and buffer you against whatever stress you may encounter. When you are ready, resume the Good Mood Diet where you left off.

DIAGNOSING THE PROBLEM

As you know from the 12-week guide, you should weigh yourself on the same day of the week at approximately the same time. After the first 4 weeks, you may choose to weigh yourself more often than once a week, possibly even daily, to keep yourself on track.

You can diagnose a problem if you:

■ Do not lose any weight for 2 consecutive weeks

■ Lose less than 0.5 kg (1 lb) a week in 2 consecutive weeks

■ Gain weight each week for 2 consecutive weeks

There is a 2-week wait because sometimes the scales gives a false impression. It can show you gaining weight if you ate salty foods the day before. Women gain water weight before their periods start. Perhaps the day before was very hot and you drank more water than usual. This may show up as water weight, too.

If you ate a lot of high-fibre, bulky foods for 1 or 2 days before the weigh-in, the scales can reflect that as well. Or, if you ate dinner very late the night before, the scale may mirror what your body is still processing, not what is in your fat cells. However, if the scales continue to show no loss for 2 weeks in a row or if you gained weight, the weight is unlikely to be due to the reasons just mentioned.

You may think that you know why you added weight and that you don't need help. Think again and step back to see the big picture.

Frank, a 55-year-old client, gained 3.2 kg (7 lb) after eating his way through a 10-day cruise.

'I planned to eat whatever I wanted,' he explained. 'I intended to get my money's worth out of that cruise. I knew I would gain weight. So what?'

In response, we pointed out that he had also paid for the Good Mood Diet. His onboard eating marathon prevented him from, in his words, 'getting his money's worth' out of the diet. The cruise offered an almost endless variety of other activities, also prepaid, that he had not taken advantage of, such as the fully equipped gym, pool, walking tours on the island destinations, and morning walks around the decks.

What else was going on, he was asked, that made eating so important? Finally he admitted that he hated going on cruises and the only reason he went was because his wife pressured him into it. His wife's sister and husband went, too.

'My wife is always after me to lose weight. I knew it would annoy her to see me ruin my diet, so I did. Besides, I can't stand my sister-in-law and her boring husband, and I didn't want to travel with them. Indulging every appetite whim was my covert way of getting back at all of them. But all I ended up doing was sabotaging myself.'

As you read through the following list of reasons weight loss can stall, keep in mind that more than one reason may be contributing to your difficulty with losing more weight.

REASONS WHY YOU ARE NOT LOSING WEIGHT

Read through the following list of problems and suggested solutions. Then, if applicable, reread the recommended pages to address your problem in detail.

Reason: Decreased or No Exercise

Explanation: Exercise is crucial for steady weight loss because it uses up calories. Most lifestyles are too sedentary to include sufficient exercise as you go about your daily activities. If you doubt this, figure out how many minutes a day you spend in physical activity. To lose weight continually, you must combine aerobic workouts with muscle strengthening. This will promote the fastest shedding of weight. Also, although you may be exercising, you may not be changing your routine. Sometimes awakening inactive muscles by changing the kind of exercise you do increases energy output. See Chapter 7 for help in developing a realistic exercise regime.

Reason: Increased Intake of High-Calorie Beverages

Explanation: Juice, fizzy drinks, coffee with sugar or cream, and alcohol can add hundreds of excess calories. Substitute zero-calorie flavoured sparkling or plain water and diet drinks for calorie-laden beverages.

Reason: Overeating at Meals

Explanation: There are a number of reasons why you might overeat at mealtime.

Not measuring portion sizes Estimating, rather than measuring, the amount of food you serve usually results in eating too much. At home, serve yourself the amount of food you think you should be eating and then, before eating, weigh or measure it. You may find that there is a big difference between how much you think you are eating and the actual amount. The difference will prevent you from losing weight consistently. Make sure you regularly measure and weigh your food.

Eating restaurant portions Most restaurants serve too-large portions of food (unless the food is very expensive, and then the portions are often tiny). Eat no more than one-half to two-thirds of a serving. Steer clear of restaurants that are infamous for serving big portions. You will end up eating too much.

Eating at prepaid buffets Avoid these if possible. If you can't skip them, stick to salads and foods that are not sauced, marinated, mixed with mayonnaise or covered with anything melted.

Not snacking on schedule If the interval between a snack and the next meal is unexpectedly stretched out, eat another small carbohydrate snack, like a slice of bread or some cereal. It is best to snack 30 to 60 minutes before the meal.

Changing medication A change in your antidepressant or mood-stabilizing medication may temporarily cause an appetite increase. Go back to phase 1 of the weight-loss plan until your appetite stabilizes. Starting medication that has weight-gain potential might also account for an unexpected halt to your weight loss.

Skipping meals When you skip a meal, you are likely to overeat at the next meal. Hunger may make you swallow your food too quickly and eat too much, often eating until your stomach feels stuffed.

Drinking alcohol In addition to adding calories to your daily intake, alcoholic drinks decrease your ability to control your eating. Keep alcohol consumption to one or two drinks a week. We found that eating a carbohydrate snack before an event at which you might drink really reduces the desire for alcohol.

Not paying attention Multi-tasking when you are eating can cause you to eat too much. This is particularly true if you are conducting business, finishing up a piece of work or talking on the telephone. When you do not notice what you are eating, you may automatically finish whatever is on the plate.

Your mother It is not necessary to clear your plate because someone is starving somewhere in the world. Serve yourself less food and give the money you save on food bills to charity.

Relatives Despite their protestations to the contrary, you will not waste away if you do not have seconds at a family gathering.

Boredom at dinner meetings Food will not render the after-dinner speaker more interesting or your table companions less tedious. Leave the table if you are bored. The 'I must make a call' excuse is always accepted.

It tastes good It is tempting to eat too much because the first few bites taste so delicious. But the last bite rarely tastes as good as the first, so you might as well save the calories.

Being a food hostage There are times when no diet-appropriate food is available. Meetings, exhibits, weddings, wakes, birthday parties, graduation dinners – the list goes on. When you find yourself in these situations, eat whatever foods seem to be relatively low in calories and avoid the obviously high-calorie choices. If you know ahead of time that there will be little that you can eat, bring food along or try to eat before you go to the event.

Reason: You Eat Too Much When It Is Time to Snack

Explanation: There are a number of reasons why you might overeat snacks.

Substituting a snack for a meal Skipping breakfast, delaying lunch or eating late dinners can make you very hungry in the late morning or late afternoon. Consequently, you may be substituting your snack for a missed meal and thus eating too much. Do not skip meals or delay them. See Chapter 5.

Snacks taste too good Selecting snacks because they taste so good will almost certainly cause you to overeat them.

Not premeasuring snacks You can eat too much of anything, even rice cakes, if you do not pay attention to the amount that should be consumed. Unless you're willing to count the number of crackers, or measure the weight of cereal or pretzels, stick with packaged snacks that have approximately the recommended amount of carbohydrate and calories. Keep away from snacks that provide two servings in one wrapper – the temptation to eat the second serving could be too strong.

Bingeing on snacks If you decrease your carbohydrate intake for any reason, you may be susceptible to bingeing when you start eating the snacks again. Follow phase 1 of the diet plan for a week to increase your serotonin quickly.

Premenstrual syndrome The mood and appetite changes that occur toward the end of the menstrual cycle can make a woman vulnerable to bingeing. If this is a problem, follow phase 1 of the diet plan on the days when you experience PMS.

Winter blues, or seasonal affective disorder (SAD) This condition causes mood changes and overeating during the dark days of autumn and winter. You may find yourself overeating snacks as the days grow shorter. Follow phase 2 of the diet plan during the weeks you suffer from the lack of sunshine. Depending on where you live and how often the sky is overcast even during the spring and summer, you may be in this phase for several months.

Other reasons A change in your medication, stress, fatigue, lack of sleep, too much work or difficulty with children can cause you to keep putting food in your mouth even though you have eaten enough. Check page 66 for a list of snacks that are rarely if ever overeaten. Also be sure to measure your snacks ahead of time. An open bag or box of snacks is an open invitation to eat too much.

Reason: Overeating in General

At times it may seem impossible to stay on the diet. When this happens, pause your weight-loss timetable until you are able to resume the diet. But it is really important to understand what caused you to stop dieting to make sure it doesn't get in the way in the future.

Life interfering with your diet plans results in eating too much. The most common causes are listed below.

No time Being unable to find time to plan for, shop for, prepare and eat the meals and snacks on the programme is one of the most common reasons people fail on any diet. Plan your eating schedule for the day while you are engaged in a routine activity like brushing your teeth or putting on makeup. Look at your weekly calendar and set aside time to go to the supermarket, cook or buy Good Mood Diet-appropriate meals and, of course, exercise. You don't have to give up sleep or your day job to do this. Like anything that is done routinely, the more you do it, the less time it takes. See Chapter 3 for suggestions.

Too much time Eating to fill empty time is a common cause of diet failure. The meals and snacks are designed to satisfy hunger and appetite. If you find yourself still looking for something to eat, ask yourself if you are really looking for something to do. See Chapter 3 and the 12-week guide for suggestions on how to replace eating with pleasurable activities that don't involve food.

Eating automatically Putting food in your mouth in response to any stress is a reflex that is hard to break. Because this eating is so unconscious, often it is not even noticed until a considerable amount of food has been consumed. If this happens, follow the first phase of the diet plan until the situation that triggered the eating is more manageable. The increase in serotonin will shut off your appetite. See Chapter 6.

Changing your routine Any diet that is followed for more than a few days is going to come up against situations that threaten the established eating and exercise routine. Travel, holidays, social and family events and houseguests can make it hard to eat diet-appropriate meals and snacks. You may not lose weight on schedule as a result, but do not allow these events to cause you to gain weight. If you have time to plan ahead before the change in routine, think about what you can eat and how to avoid fattening foods. You may find that taking foods with you on a trip will help you stay on the diet. See Chapter 8.

Feeling deprived because you are dieting The Good Mood Diet is designed to make you feel satisfied and content with what you are eating, even if the foods are not those you would choose to eat if you were not dieting. If you feel deprived, it may be because food was acting as a substitute for other things that are missing in your life. This is very common. Look over Chapter 3 and the 12-week guide for suggestions for making other aspects of your life as fulfilling as food once was.

Shift work and jet lag Forcing your body to awaken and sleep at abnormal times often results in eating to fall asleep and to stay awake. Neither works. Avoid eating heavy meals and drinking alcohol before you go to sleep. Use exercise rather than food to make your body stay awake when it would rather not.

False hunger signals An acidic stomach, which can be caused by many medications, reflux or other disorders, can mimic hunger. If you feel hunger at inappropriate times, such as an hour after a meal, try antacid to see if the feeling goes away. Also check with your doctor.

Lack of sleep Mood changes and fatigue induced by lack of sleep can lead to overeating and make it harder to stay on the Good Mood Diet. Getting enough sleep will help you lose weight.

GET A GOOD NIGHT'S SLEEP

Try these suggestions:

- Avoid caffeine after 2 p.m.
- Be sure your bedroom is calm, pleasant and free of clutter.
- Use your bedroom only for sleeping, reading and intimate activities.
- Keep the temperature cool but not cold.
- Invest in a good mattress; you spend one-third of your day on it.
- Go to bed and get up at the same time every day.
- Follow a before-bed ritual, which may include doing some gentle stretches, listening to calming music, reading a relaxing book, or soaking in a soothing bath.
- Do not exercise within 3 hours of your bedtime. Exercise is a good antidote to sleepiness; the increased blood flow will make you feel more awake.
- Do not drink alcohol within 2 hours of your bedtime.

FREQUENTLY ASKED QUESTIONS

Will eating late at night cause me to gain weight?

No, it won't, unless you consume more calories than permitted on the diet plan. In the UK and US, late-night eating is not regarded as diet-friendly. That may be because most people who eat at that time do one of two things, and sometimes both. Starved because they haven't gotten enough food earlier in the day, they consume too many calories. Or, as they sit in front of the TV, they mindlessly stuff themselves with large quantities of junk food.

In contrast, look at countries like Spain or Argentina, where dinner traditionally starts at 10 or 11 p.m. Despite this late meal, those countries have lower obesity rates.

I love juice and now I realize that my weight loss has slowed down because I drink so many glasses. But my medication makes me thirsty and juice is the only thing that satisfies it. What can I do?

You might try adding a splash of juice to flavoured carbonated water. You could also drink a zero-calorie, fruit-flavoured drink or keep water in a jug in the refrigerator with a slice or two of fresh orange, lime or lemon added to it. Citrus-infused water is an effective way to satisfy your thirst.

Can't I indulge in a fancy coffee drink?

If you neglect to factor in the calorie content of beverages, you'll end up thirsty for weight loss. Consider that coffee or tea with large amounts of whole milk or cream and 'speciality' coffees spiked with syrups and topped with whipped cream can pack 400 or more calories. Additionally, sugar-laden fizzy drinks and juices all add unwanted calories. Unless you are willing to count the beverage as part of your meal or snack (such as juice, a fat-free latte, or a protein smoothie), drink water, diet soft drinks or other calorie-free beverages. We encourage you to consume as many calorie-free drinks as you like.

Maintaining Your Weight Loss

The weight is gone. Your body is in better shape than it has ever been. You now understand how to use serotonin-producing foods to activate your eating and mood control systems. As you continue exercising to build muscle mass and improve your stamina, you feel fit and energetic and look terrific. And of course you want to stay that way.

But how do you do it? How do you go from eating fewer calories in order to lose weight to eating the right amount to maintain weight? How do you go from exercising to lose weight to doing enough to remain fit?

You do it gently. Your body and your mind need time to adjust to the change from weight loss to weight maintenance. It is like installing a new system that regulates the temperature in your home. It takes a while before you know at what temperature to set the thermostat to get the room temperature you want, regardless of whether it is very cold or very hot outside.

In a similar way, when you are on the Good Mood Diet your body is in weight-loss mode and your mind is in control. If you flip over to a 'now the diet is over and I can eat whatever I want' mindset, you will be in danger of gaining weight very quickly.

The good news is that you are now thinner. The not-so-good news is that your body does not require as many calories to maintain your thinner size. For instance, if you started the diet at 82 kg (12 st 9 lb) and now you weigh 75.5 kg (11 st 4 lb), you now need fewer calories to support your lighter body.

So you must carefully and slowly adjust your intake of calories to meet your new body's requirements. Make sure you do not overshoot or undershoot the amount of food your body requires to maintain your goal weight.

YOUR BRAIN IS YOUR MAINTENANCE BUDDY

Regardless of your lower weight, your brain will continue to demand serotonin. As long as you feed it what it needs, your brain will work with you, moderating your appetite, upholding your good mood and subduing cravings. So you must continue to snack in serotonin-friendly ways.

Follow the snack size recommendations given below and eat the snack in the late afternoon, since that is when serotonin levels seem lowest. If you find that your body now responds better to snacking at another time of the day, then switch to the most effective time.

In the maintenance phase, snacks for men and women should contain the following:

- Carbohydrate: 25 to 30 grams
- Fat: 2 to 3 grams (avoid trans fat)
- Protein: no more than 5 grams
- Calories: no more than 140 calories

Your choices can come from the list provided for phase 3 (see page 67). However, there are new snack options coming into our supermarkets all the time and if they fit the portion sizes, do give them a try.

If necessary, your snack intake can be increased to two a day. You know the signs: cravings for carbohydrate, not feeling satisfied or contented after eating, moodiness and restlessness. Continue on an increased snack regime until you feel your serotonin eating-control system is working and your mood is under control. Then switch back to eating one snack a day.

If you find yourself eating after dinner, go back immediately to eating the phase 1 dinners to raise your serotonin levels between dinner and bedtime. Make sure to distinguish between feeling a need to snack because your dinner was not satisfying and feeling a need to snack because you are not satisfied with your life.

Stress, especially if it is chronic, has the potential to erode your serotonin levels and ultimately your control over your food intake. Joan's story is an example of how to deal with such a situation.

A year after Joan had successfully lost more than 22.6 kg (3½ st) she called to check in. She told us she had started eating two snacks each day because her cravings had come back, with good reason.

'I need the snacks now more than ever,' she said. 'My father suffered several strokes, and he is no longer able to live on his own. But he refuses to go into an assisted-living facility. So in addition to working full-time, I am trying to take care of him in the evenings. I crave carbohydrates all the time because I am so stressed. But I haven't gained back any weight, and I can count on the snacks to help me feel calm and get me to sleep.'

We suggested that she might want to eat a protein-free dinner so she would feel relaxed when she took care of her father in the evenings.

That's just what Joan did. 'It still amazes me how making such a little change in my eating can make such a big difference in my emotional life as well as my weight,' she told us.

SETTING YOUR NEW EATING AND EXERCISE THERMOSTAT

When you feel that it is too hot or cold in a room, you check the temperature gauge on the thermostat. When you want to know whether your level of eating and exercise is appropriate for maintenance, you weigh yourself. Only the scales will tell you how you are doing.

After you complete the 12-week plan, give yourself 4 weeks to determine what your calorie and exercise levels should be to maintain your weight. Do not rush this process. During this time you will be systematically testing how much more you can eat and how much exercise you should be doing to keep your weight stable. It is important that you make only one change at a time over a 2-week period, either in how much you eat or how much you exercise. That way you can track the impact each change has on your weight.

The time will pass quickly because you will be occupied with hearing how terrific you look, as well as with trying on new clothes.

Weeks 1 and 2

Weigh yourself daily during the first 2 weeks. If you cannot weigh yourself every day, then do so as frequently as possible.

Add 200 calories to the phase 3 eating plan and continue to snack every afternoon on the maintenance snacks. The extra calories do not represent much food. For example, they equal a couple of glasses of wine, 2 tablespoons of salad dressing or peanut butter, or a small dessert. Keeping a food diary will help you monitor your eating.

Do not change your exercise routine. If you decrease your exercise during this time and you find yourself gaining weight, you will not know whether it is due to eating slightly more or using fewer calories with activity.

If you find yourself still losing weight at the end of the 2 weeks, do not change your eating again until you test the effect of altering your exercise regime on your weight loss.

If you have gained weight at the end of the 2 weeks, continue on the phase 3 eating plan and cut out the additional 200 calories a day. If you added more than 200 calories a day during this time, then you are not really testing what you should be eating during maintenance. Go back to phase 2 for a week and follow it with phase 3 until you get to your starting maintenance weight. Then you can try again to add 200 calories a day for 2 weeks.

Weeks 3 and 4

Weigh yourself every 3 or 4 days, although you can continue to weigh yourself daily if you prefer.

During these 2 weeks you will see what effect decreasing your exercise level has on your weight. If you are committed to continuing your exercise routine, then skip this test period. But if you are honest with yourself and admit that despite your best intentions you will not continue to do the workout routine you undertook during the weight-loss period, this is the time to see what it will do to your weight. Do not change your eating at this time. Remember: you cannot change two things at once.

Adjusting your eating and exercise thermostat after these test weeks depends on how your body responds to slightly increasing calories and decreasing exercise.

Pick a routine you think you will stick with over the long haul and start to follow it.

If, at the end of 4 weeks, your weight did not change, you are in maintenance. Do not increase your calorie intake. Be vigilant about portion sizes and fat intake.

If your weight decreased, you can gently add another 100 to 200 calories to your daily food intake and keep your exercise intensity and frequency constant. Then, see what your weight is after another 2 weeks. When it is stable, stay with that number of calories and that exercise routine, which you have fine-tuned for your body.

If your weight increases by 0.5–1 kg (1–2 lb), it means that you cannot reduce your exercise while you add a small number of daily calories. Bring your exercise back to the level that allowed you to lose weight. If you do not, then the weight will eventually start to creep back on.

Note: If you gained more than 2.2 kg (5 lb), go back on the diet for a month or until you lose the weight again. Follow phase 2 for 1 week and then, if you feel that you are in control, switch to phase 3. Here's a useful reminder: an increase of 4.5 kg (10 lb) equals a bigger clothing size.

After the first 4 weeks, you can continue to test your body to see what happens when calories and/or exercise change. You may find that a period of increased activity allows you to eat substantially more without gaining weight. For example, many clients who go on a holiday walk so much that they can enjoy the culinary delights of the location without gaining weight.

On the other hand, seasonal changes may, without your realizing it, decrease your activity. A long, rainy winter or hot, humid summer can keep you inside or force you to use the car rather than your feet for errands. This simple change in activity can reduce your body's need for calories and, unless you are aware of it, can spur a small weight gain. If this happens, rather than eating less in response, find some way to increase your exercise.

CONTINUE TO EXERCISE

Keeping active to maintain weight loss is the big lesson that Jim, a client, discovered. A professor at a university, he always lost weight on other diet plans and then gained it back within months of ending the regime. But after using the Good Mood Diet programme and losing more than 32 kg (5 st), he was determined to remain thin. Once he began maintenance he was surprised at how finely tuned his body was to changes in his food intake and exercise.

'I finally realized that I had to be engaged in consistent physical activity at least three times a week,' he said. 'One of the added benefits of the diet programme is that I became used to exercising. When I don't do it I feel sluggish, which I don't like.'

Donna, another determined dieter who shed over 20 kg (3¼ st) in 6 months, discovered that maintenance led to new interests. 'There's nothing I like better than taking my kids to the zoo, but before the diet programme I would always get tired out before they did,' she told us on a follow-up visit. 'But after I lost a few pounds and began walking daily, I could start to keep up with them. After I lost the weight I took training at the zoo and now I'm a tour guide. Every time I walk through there I'm reminded of what I've achieved. The workers at the zoo keep asking me how I lost the weight. I'm glad to share the information because it reinforces my own commitment to staying thin and active.'

Tip: As soon as you reach your weight goal, buy a new size of clothing and donate the rest. Doing so will motivate you to maintain what you've achieved.

Do continue to challenge yourself with new activities to exercise different muscles and alleviate boredom. You still may never love exercise. Nonetheless, let the many benefits you gain be the encouragement that keeps you physically active. Increasing your exercise level is always an option for enjoyment or to achieve a particular goal, like walking in a 10-K fundraising event.

Keep in mind that, for weight-loss maintenance and overall health, more is not necessarily better. Build up the intensity of your activities slowly and listen to your body for any signs of overuse injury, such as persistent joint or muscle pain, excessive fatigue, headaches, insomnia, bowel irregularities or malaise. If you have any reason for concern, check with your health-care provider for fitness guidance.

MAINTENANCE = ADJUSTMENT

One client, Meredith, who lost 13.6 kg (2¼ st), said that maintenance is all about keeping her lost weight off no matter what else is going on in her life.

'When I don't have time to go to the gym I try to get in some exercise at work, like always taking the stairs instead of the lift. To break up my exercise routine I go to a Latin dance class; it's a real energy booster. And when those stress levels surge I practise relaxation techniques every few hours.

'To de-stress, I also like a gentle yoga class, even if it means skipping the calorie-burning aerobics class. And I know that the snack I carry in my bag is ready if I feel really stressed.

'If I gain weight, I immediately go back to phase 2. With my two snacks a day and carbohydrate plus a little protein for dinner, I feel satisfied and avoid eating at night. Plus it's a whole lot easier to take off a few pounds than 20.

'I also plan unstructured time, when I fit in nonessentials that nonetheless are still important to me. Talking on the phone with friends, browsing at the bookshop because I feel like it, or just relaxing matter. But I also give myself rewards for staying on track. Before the diet I used food as a reward, but now my treats are theatre tickets and shoes.'

STAY ON COURSE

That's what Nicole, a client who dropped 9 kg (1½ st), did. A full-time mother of two small children, she also juggled a career conducted from home. Add to that a husband who travelled frequently for work. Consequently, her schedule changed from day to day, as did demands on her time.

Therefore, she planned ahead for exercise, trips to the supermarket with her kids, and evenings enjoying a movie with her husband.

But one day her well-thought-out arrangements went awry. 'My reward for maintaining my weight loss is to book a haircut and high-lights, along with a pedicure, at a salon every 8 weeks. Then I take a yoga class nearby. I hire a babysitter and I know that the next few hours belong to me,' Nicole related.

'But one day my standing appointments were not in the book. Nor were there any openings, and there wasn't a yoga class for several hours. Instead of wasting time complaining to the manager, I figured that there were other ways to pamper myself.

'I returned to my car, grabbed the running shoes, tracksuit bottoms and T-shirt that I keep there, changed clothes at the hairdresser's, and then drove to a nearby park and went jogging. Afterward, I retrieved my mat from the car, spread it out under a tree and did a half hour of yoga. I still had time for a leisurely lunch before the babysitter was due to leave. I call this my Plan B, since the well-thought-out Plan A fell apart. I didn't let the disruption ruin my day. Instead, I adapted to it and ended up enjoying a very pleasant interlude.'

THE NINE RULES OF SUCCESSFUL MAINTENANCE

1. Don't let deviations become derailments. If your eating or exer-cise begins to veer off track, don't throw in the towel and give it all up. Re-establish your good weight-loss habits quickly, before the small weight gain becomes unmanageable.

2. Don't beat yourself up for gaining weight. Take the opportunity to learn what didn't work, recommit and get a fresh start. You know what to do.

3. If you want to indulge in a high calorie meal or treat, make it a conscious decision. Do it with your eyes open. There is no such thing as a deviation if it is done with control and choice. You must take charge. If you plan for deviations, you will maintain control and be able to get back on track.

4. When you are tempted to stop exercising or planning your meals or you forget to snack, remind yourself of what you have gained by losing weight and use the benefits as motivation.

5. Don't lose sight of your accomplishments. Look in the mirror.

6. Reward yourself as you maintain the eating, exercise and mental habits you established. Buy fresh flowers every week, socialize with friends, schedule child-care cover so you can spend time alone with your spouse or partner, or book an outdoor holiday that takes advantage of your new stamina and energy. Do whatever brings you joy.

7. Keep tabs on yourself. That means weighing yourself on a regular basis. Keep a food diary, or choose an article of clothing that fit when you reached your weight-loss goal and try it on weekly.

8. Monitor your portion sizes every 2 or 3 weeks. Before sitting down to eat, take a minute to see how much food you put on your plate. Is there enough protein, too much pasta, too few vegetables? If you are moving away from the portion sizes that got and kept you thin, go back to them.

9. Don't deprive yourself of higher-calorie or higher-fat foods that you enjoy. But do eat those foods in moderation and watch the scales to limit any damage.

MAINTAIN THE BALANCE YOU'VE ACHIEVED

It's easy to revert to old, unhealthy eating habits and discontinue exercise when stressful events happen. Many events can overtake your time, emotions and lifestyle.

That's what happened to Jane, a 70-plus-year-old client who had lost about 9.9 kg (1½ st) on the diet. A regular at her health club until her daughter's diagnosis of breast cancer and subsequent surgery, Jane gained back nearly half the weight she had lost. While she did not have time to see us, we did speak via phone. When we tried to convince her that her own health required her to eat healthily and continue to exercise, she became angry and said that she could not be concerned about caring for herself when her daughter needed her.

After things calmed down and we could talk face-to-face, Jane admitted that she could have chosen to eat the correct foods, both in the hospital cafeteria and at her daughter's house. She did have the time to go to the gym in the morning before going to see her daughter because her son-in-law was home.

When asked why she didn't take care of herself she replied, 'Because I felt guilty that I was healthy and she was not. I just couldn't do anything to make myself even healthier. When I started to gain back the weight, I sort of felt that I was being punished because my daughter was sick and I wasn't.'

Realizing that stress was undermining her life, Jane resumed the diet and went back to the gym. 'Being healthy for my daughter, and myself,' she realized, 'is the best thing I can do'.

YOUR MAINTENANCE CHECKLIST

1. Incorporate the principles and parameters of the 12-week guide into your calendar or diary. Use whatever tools you need to maintain your awareness of the Good Mood Diet. Forming a plan, tracking weight-loss progress and acknowledging success at keeping weight off all work.

2. Plan meals and snacks ahead of time when possible. Correct portion sizes are essential, so keeping a food diary is a helpful aid.

3. Keep fat content low when you are cooking and when you are dining out (for example, watch out for salad dressings, butter on rolls and so on).

4. Weigh yourself at least once a week.

5. Do some kind of exercise every day. Mix it up. Walk one day, use weights on another, attend a dance class on a third. Do what interests you.

6. Schedule personal time.

PART FOUR

COOKING THE

GOOD MOOD DIET

CHAPTER TWELVE

The Kitchen List for a Meal in Minutes

Your kitchen is your best friend when you are hungry and you don't want to spend time and effort cooking a meal for yourself, and your family, to eat. So we've put together a list for ideally stocking a kitchen. With these items on hand, you won't be forced to run to the supermarket when you are starving, much less rely on a meal in a box or a takeaway container.

All friendships are very personal, so fill your kitchen with the foods and equipment that meet your specific needs. To make life easier, store the food and equipment in places where you can reach what you need without resorting to climbing a stepladder.

For quick meals, keep these foods in the freezer:

Chicken breasts or mini fillets

Cold deli meats (ham, roast beef, turkey) wrapped in lunch-size
    quantities

Fruit, such as berries (not in syrup)

Prawns, shelled

Salmon fillets

Scallops

Vegetables (asparagus, broccoli, brussels sprouts, cauliflower,
    mushrooms, peas, peppers, spinach, squash)

Veggie burgers and sausages

For quick meals, keep these foods in the pantry:

Apple sauce

Barbecue sauce

Beans, canned (baked, black, chickpeas, kidney, white)

Bread, wholemeal and multigrain, including pitta

Breadcrumbs

Cereals

Cranberries, dried

Fish, canned (salmon and tuna packed in water)

Herbs and spices, dried (basil, cinnamon, curry powder, Italian
seasoning, nutmeg, oregano, tarragon, thyme etc.)

Hoisin sauce

Jam or marmalade

Ketchup

Mustard

Noodles

Oil, olive, rapeseed and sesame

Pasta (any varieties)

Peppercorns

Raisins and sultanas

Red peppers, roasted (jarred)

Rice, brown and white

Salsa (tomato)

Salt

Soups, low-fat and low-sodium, packet or canned

Soy sauce or tamari, low-sodium

Teriyaki sauce

Tomato sauce, fat-free or low-fat

Vinegar, balsamic

Worcestershire sauce

For quick meals, keep these foods in the refrigerator:

Cheese, grated, low-fat

Cheese slices, low-fat

Cottage cheese, fat-free or low-fat, plain, with pineapple

Eggs

Feta cheese

Fruit juice

Fresh fruit (apples, apricots, berries, citrus fruits, melons and pears or other seasonal fruit like peaches and plums)*

Fresh vegetables (broccoli, cabbage, carrots, courgettes, cucumbers, fennel, leeks, mushrooms, onions, radishes, spring onions, sugar snap peas, sweet peppers, tomatoes)

Garlic

Ginger

Milk, skimmed or semi-skimmed

Parmesan cheese, grated

Polenta, ready-made

Ricotta cheese, low-fat

Salad dressing, fat-free and low-fat

Salad, prewashed, such as baby spinach, cabbage, romaine, salad mixture

Soya milk, fat-free or low-fat, chocolate, plain or vanilla

Tortillas (corn and wheat)

Yogurt, flavoured, fat-free

Yogurt, natural, fat-free or low-fat

For quick snacks, keep these foods in the freezer:

Ice cream, low-fat

Sorbets and frozen fruit bars

The Skinny Cow frozen desserts

Yogurt, frozen, fat-free

*Bananas should be kept outside of refrigerator

For quick snacks, keep these foods in the pantry:

Cereals, cold and instant oats

Crackers, fat-free or low-fat

Hot chocolate mix, fat-free

Japanese rice crackers

Marshmallow Fluff

Marshmallows

Muesli/cereal bars, low-fat

Popcorn, air-popped

Rice cakes, plain and sweetened

For quick snacks, keep these foods in the refrigerator:

English muffins, pitta, sliced bread*

Fat-free crème fraîche

*Multigrain and wholemeal. Look for varieties that do not have 'unbleached flour' or wheat flour as the first ingredient.

RECOMMENDED APPLIANCES

- Food processor
- Handheld blender
- Kitchen scales
- Measuring spoons
- Mini grill
- Rice cooker
- Steamer

CHAPTER THIRTEEN

Basic Meals and Quick Kitchen Tricks

If you have little or no time or desire to cook, this chapter is for you. Our clients who do not like to cook found it was really easy to follow the Good Mood Diet programme using these quick tricks.

BASIC BREAKFAST

Breakfast consists of protein, carbohydrate and a piece of fruit or fruit juice. If you prefer, you can eat or drink your fruit serving at another time of day – just be sure that you don't count it as a snack.

1. Protein

2. Carbohydrate

3. Fruit or fruit juice

Breakfast Extras

These flavourful add-ons contain few calories but give food another taste dimension.

1 wedge Laughing Cow Light cheese; mix with scrambled eggs or use as a spread on bread

½ slice low-fat cheese slices or mozzarella; mix with eggs

1 generous teaspoon jam

1 generous teaspoon honey

1 tablespoon salsa

1 thin slice low-fat ham

2 slices soya 'bacon'; crumble into scrambled eggs

Chopped onion, pepper, mushroom

GRAB-AND-GO BREAKFAST

A protein bar containing 200 to 300 calories with 10 grams of protein for women and 15 grams of protein for men, along with a fruit, is an adequate substitute for a sit-down meal. Guess what? A fast-food sandwich of egg on a bagel or an English muffin with a small juice is also acceptable. Do not include breakfast meat or cheese on the sandwich.

BASIC LUNCH

At its most basic, lunch consists of three elements: protein, vegetables and a dressing to liven things up. An enormous variety of fat-free and low-fat salad dressings, salsas, mustards, chutneys and hot sauces is available. Use 2 tablespoons, along with dried herbs and spices, as you like to dress up salads or vegetables. They can also be used to perk up protein and carbohydrate dishes.

1. Protein

  Phase 1:

  Women: 115 g (4 oz)

  Men: 170 g (6 oz)

  Phases 2 and 3:

  Women: 90 g (3 oz)

  Men: 145 g (5 oz)

2. Vegetables, at least 150–200 g (5½–7 oz), raw or cooked

3. Dressing, 2 tablespoons

Lunch Suggestions

If you always wait until your evening meal to eat protein, you may not know how to add this essential nutrient to your lunch. It is easier than you think, even if you take your lunch in a sandwich box rather than buying a hot meal.

Salad bars are good places to look for protein (along with those veggies you should be eating). You will find cottage cheese, plain tuna, lean cold meats, tofu and hard-boiled eggs. Since it is difficult to judge the quantity of protein you should be eating, put the protein in a separate container and weigh it if possible.

You can increase the protein content of your meal by adding hard-boiled egg whites. Throw away the egg yolks, which contain all the fat and most of the calories, and eat the cooked whites. (This is the hard-boiled version of an egg-white omelette.) Since egg whites are so low in calories and high in protein, you can add two or three to whatever protein you are eating. Stuff some of the tuna salad into the egg white and enjoy a yolk-free deviled egg.

If you prefer to eat a vegetarian source of protein, there are many soya-protein-based foods that require relatively little time to prepare. Just as you do with other packaged foods, check the nutrition label to make sure that the major ingredient is protein, not fat or carbohydrate.

Soya content can vary widely. Don't be fooled into thinking that just because a product is vegetarian, it is high in protein. Check the labels carefully.

If you want to bring lunch from home, you can buy prepared chicken, prawns, beef and fish at your supermarket, along with a wide selection of salads and vegetables from the salad bar. One of our clients told us that when she bought cold meats from the deli counter she asked for several packages weighing about 100 g (3½ oz) each and froze what she did not use right away.

If you cook protein foods for other people to enjoy at dinner, prepare a lunch-size portion for yourself to eat the next day. Just be sure that you, and not someone else in the family, get to eat it.

If possible, make lunch a hot meal. Tuna and cottage cheese can become very boring very quickly. Check out the lunch selections at restaurants close to work and review Chapter 8 for suggested menu choices. Don't be shy about requesting extra protein if the serving is small, and don't hesitate to ask how many grams are in a serving. All restaurants know exactly how much they are serving. It is figured into their pricing and inventory control.

Also, let the season guide you in what you have for lunch. A bowl of

GRAB-AND-GO LUNCH

If you have no time to prepare or buy lunch, take a pouch of tuna (some are already seasoned), some cherry tomatoes and baby carrots, and a plastic fork and a napkin with you when you leave the house.

Protein bars with at least 20 grams of protein for women and 25 to 30 grams of protein for men and no more than 5 or 6 grams of fat, paired with fruit or vegetables, are a last-resort substitute for a traditional lunch. Add milk or low-fat yogurt to increase the protein.

If you exercise at lunchtime and don't have time for a regular meal, shakes with similar amounts of protein are also acceptable. Toss a bag of baby carrots or a can of V8 or tomato juice into your gym bag. That way you'll get some veggies along with your protein. Make sure that you choose the low-sodium varieties. Excess sodium leads to water retention. If you cannot get vegetables, choose a piece of fruit instead.

hot soup brimming with chunks of chicken or hearty beef stew tastes wonderful on a cold day in February. A crisp salad with marinated prawns or fish grilled the night before is a delight on a hot summer day. (Remember to use a chill box when the weather is warm.)

If you eat lunch at home, make sure you take the time to prepare something for yourself. Your 3-year-old's leftovers should not be your midday meal.

BASIC DINNER

The basic dinner consists of carbohydrates and vegetables in phase 1 and of protein, carbohydrates and vegetables in phases 2 and 3. A good dressing can do wonders for any meal. See pages 254 to 257 in Chapter 14 for some easy and fast homemade dressings.

1. Protein

Phase 1:

None

Phases 2 and 3:

Women: 60 g (2 oz)

Men: 115 g (4 oz)

2. Carbohydrate

3. Vegetables, at least 150–200 g (5½–7 oz), raw or cooked

4. Dressing, 2 tablespoons

Phase 1 Dinner Suggestions

You can have pizza for dinner, just not the kind that is topped with four different kinds of cheese and a layer of pepperoni. Pizza that has little or no cheese and lots of tomato sauce and vegetables is a fine dinner choice. The label will tell you how much you can have. Women should eat about 350 calories of pizza and men 450 calories to get the right amount of carbohydrates.

Is a large bowl of mashed potatoes your idea of the ultimate comfort food? Now you can have it. Just be sure you soften the potato with stock rather than with butter and cream.

Phase 2 Dinner Suggestions

Don't like to cook? Here are some simple tips for a fast, nutritious meal that you can make in minutes.

- Buy roasted chicken or turkey breast and add a couple of ounces of it, along with frozen vegetables, to prepared low-fat chicken soup with noodles.
- Add cooked chicken and vegetables to rice you cooked and froze in plastic bags earlier in the week. Microwave the rice for 5 minutes to heat it.
- Add cooked chicken or canned tuna to pasta cooked ahead of time and frozen. Top with ready-made low-fat tomato sauce.
- Heat low-fat hot dogs or vegetarian sausages and baked beans together. They cook in minutes.
- Microwave ready-to-eat fresh noodles or flavoured microwave rice with cooked chicken or prawns.
- Wrap cooked chicken, rice and vegetables in a flour tortilla and add some salsa.
- Keep bagged salad greens or grated coleslaw mix handy and mix with low-calorie salad dressing for an instant side salad.

COOKING PROTEIN

Protein – beef, fish, poultry, pork and tofu – can be cooked quickly with little or no fat using the following methods.

Grill: It takes little time and the outside of the food becomes crispy.

Microwave: Especially good for fresh or frozen whitefish. Cook on High for 5 to 10 minutes. The fish stays remarkably moist.

Steam: Chicken breasts or fish will cook in about 15 minutes.

Stir-fry: Stir-fry protein in a wok on high heat with 1 to 2 tablespoons of oil to lock in flavour. Cook chopped vegetables in the same pan for an easy one-dish meal.

Tip: Speciality mustards make the protein component of any meal more flavourful without adding calories. Mustard is fat-free and comes in an amazing number of varieties. Use mustard on chicken, fish and grilled lean beef.

COOKING CARBOHYDRATES

Potatoes, pasta, rice, polenta, corn, peas, bread, tortillas, couscous: the carbohydrate list goes on and on. Our clients have said that potatoes, pasta and rice are their favourites for making quick meals. Microwave rice can be prepared in minutes; just follow the package directions. Here are some fast ways to cook potatoes, pasta and even polenta.

Potatoes

Baked potatoes, both white and sweet, are easy to prepare and delicious, especially if you vary the toppings you use from the list opposite. Check Chapter 6 for portion sizes.

Conventional Oven Baked Potato

Preheat oven to 230°C/450°F/gas 8. Pierce a washed and dried potato (white or sweet) with a sharp fork or knife and place it on a baking tray. Bake 50 to 60 minutes or until tender.

TASTY, LOW-CALORIE POTATO TOPPINGS

- 2 tablespoons low-fat soured cream or low-fat ricotta cheese per serving with snipped fresh chives
- Salsa with sliced chilli peppers
- Chopped jarred roasted red peppers with 1 teaspoon sautéed chopped garlic
- 2 tablespoons red caviar per serving with chopped spring onions
- Mushrooms sautéed with olive oil cooking spray
- 1 tablespoon low-fat grated cheese
- 1 tablespoon light cream cheese
- 1 tablespoon pesto
- 1 tablespoon horseradish cream
- 1 large red onion, chopped, cooked over very low heat for 20 minutes with 1 tablespoon olive oil plus 2 tablespoons balsamic vinegar
- 75 g (2½ oz) broccoli sautéed in 1 tablespoon olive oil with a pinch of chilli flakes and 1 clove garlic, chopped, plus 1 tablespoon low-fat grated mozzarella cheese
- 1 tablespoon crumbled bacon or bacon bits plus 2 tablespoons low-fat soured cream
- 2–3 drained marinated artichoke hearts
- 2 tablespoons chopped sun-dried tomatoes marinated in olive oil, drained
- 60 g (2 oz) baked beans or low-fat chilli

Microwave Oven Baked Potato

Pierce a washed and dried potato (white or sweet) with a sharp fork or knife and cook on High for 10 minutes or until tender when pierced with a fork, turning once during cooking. Let potato stand for 5 to 10 minutes before serving.

Combination Conventional and Microwave Oven Baked Potato

Combining cooking methods is a quick way to crisp the outside of the potato while leaving the inside soft and fluffy. Preheat the oven to 230°C/450°F/gas 8. Pierce a washed and dried potato (white or sweet) with a sharp fork or knife. Place the potato in the microwave and cook on High for 8 minutes. Then put the potato in the oven on a baking tray and bake for another 8 to 10 minutes.

Twice-Baked Potato

Preheat oven to 200°C/400°F/gas 6. Cut baked or microwaved white or sweet potato in half lengthwise. Leaving the skin intact, scoop out the inside, place the pulp in a bowl and add toppings. Mash together. Put potato mixture back in the skin. Place filled potato halves on a baking tray and bake for 10 minutes or until hot.

Pasta

To reheat leftover pasta, use the following restaurant trick: put it in a colander and place the colander in boiling water for 1 minute. Toss the pasta with any of the following ingredients. The quantities given are for 200–285 g (7–10 oz) of cooked pasta. These toppings also can be used for rice, couscous and other grains.

- 1 clove garlic, crushed and sautéed in 1 tablespoon olive oil, plus a pinch of chilli flakes and 1 teaspoon dried basil

- 230-g can crushed tomatoes with a few fresh basil leaves

- 1 tablespoon olive oil, 2 tablespoons raisins and 1 tablespoon pine nuts

- 120 ml (4 fl oz) passata with a few chopped anchovies or black olives

- 2 tablespoons freshly grated Parmesan cheese and ground black pepper to taste

- 60 g (2 oz) chopped smoked salmon and 100 g (3½ oz) steamed asparagus tips

- 1 tablespoon capers, juice from ½ lemon, 1 tablespoon olive oil and 1 teaspoon Italian seasoning

- 1 tablespoon sesame oil, 2 teaspoons light soy sauce, 2 table-spoons orange juice, 1 tablespoon rice vinegar, ½ teaspoon ground ginger and 1 clove garlic, chopped

- 1 tablespoon chopped sun-dried tomato marinated in olive oil, 1 teaspoon red wine vinegar, 1 teaspoon dried basil and a pinch of crushed chilli flakes

Basic Polenta

This cornmeal-based starch is very popular in Northern Italy. When prepared in the traditional way it requires a lot of stirring, but it cooks in minutes in a microwave.

240 ml (8 fl oz) water

30 g (1 oz) cornmeal

¼ teaspoon salt

Place ingredients together in a microwave-safe bowl. Microwave on High for 3 minutes, stirring twice. Let stand for about 4 minutes. It will become firm. If you would like it to be softer, add a little more water after removing from the microwave.

Note: Cooked polenta can be refrigerated overnight. The next day, coat a baking tray with cooking spray. Spread the polenta on the tray in a thin layer. Bake at 180°C/350°F/gas 4 for 5 to 7 minutes. The result will be a crisp, pizza-like crust.

COOKING VEGETABLES

You can always use frozen vegetables – they cook in minutes – or toss together a salad using prepackaged greens. However, if you feel like preparing fresh vegetables, here are quick and easy ways to do it.

Blanch: Add 1 teaspoon of salt to a large pot of water and bring to a rapid boil. Toss in vegetables and return to the boil. After 2 minutes, drain the vegetables in a colander and rinse with very cold water. Vegetables stay crisp, flavourful and colourful.

Grill: Spray vegetables with olive oil cooking spray or lightly brush with olive oil and place on a preheated grill rack. Cook until browned, turning once.

Microwave: Place in a microwave-safe dish along with 2 tablespoons of water, and cover. Microwave on High until the veggies are tender. Be careful when removing the cover, because the steam that escapes will be very hot.

Sauté: Heat a frying pan coated with cooking spray over medium-high heat. Add the vegetables and cook, stirring frequently, to the desired level of crispness or tenderness.

Steam: Place a steamer basket or wire rack in a large pot of water or a rice cooker. Bring to the boil over high heat. Place the veggies in the basket or rack and steam until just tender.

Vegetable Suggestions

If you rarely eat vegetables, you may look at these recommendations and say, 'No way'. But when they are prepared in interesting ways, vegetables can taste just as good as any meat-based main course. One of the best ways to try vegetables beyond a lettuce leaf and a few peas is to eat vegetable dishes at a Chinese restaurant. If you like them, order extra portions and freeze them.

Buy a variety of fresh salad ingredients from a salad bar so you can see which ones you might be willing to eat again. Combine chicken, beef, tuna or prawns with some chopped vegetables, season with a tasty dressing (see pages 254–57), and wrap the mixture in a large lettuce leaf. You can even dip the lettuce wrap in a seafood cocktail or a spicy sauce.

CHAPTER FOURTEEN

Recipes

Designed to provide a wide repertoire of salads, cooked vegetables, starches and proteins throughout all phases of the diet, the following recipes will help you create easy and enjoyable meals. Of course, you can also use your creativity to modify the recipes to suit your tastes.

To make sure that you are eating the correct amount of protein or carbohydrate, measure the ingredient amounts carefully.

The recipes provide a single serving for either a woman or a man, with the correct quantities of protein and carbohydrates for each phase of the diet. However, all recipes can be doubled or tripled to serve more people. Some recipes include suggestions for an accompanying vegetable and a low-fat dressing. You can always add vegetables prepared with no more than a teaspoon of added fat to any recipe to complete the meal. The calorie content of the recipes is in the appropriate range for you to lose weight consistently.

Because vegetables contain carbohydrate, the nutrient analyses for the lunch recipes list that value even though no starchy carbohydrates are added to the meal.

The dinners in the Serotonin Balance and Control phases may seem high in protein. This is because starchy foods, such as rice or potatoes, contain a small amount of protein. However, the protein in most carbohydrate foods lacks sufficient amounts of certain amino acids that your body needs. It is of a lower quality than animal sources of protein, like eggs, fish and meat.

For all carbohydrate ingredients like pasta, bread and rice, you can substitute whole grain varieties for added fibre and nutrients. Brown rice is a better choice than white rice for leftovers because it does not become dry or gluey. Make an extra batch and store it for another quick meal 1 or 2 days later. Brown rice also freezes well.

Finally, unlike many diet plans that reduce the number of calories in each recipe by making the serving sizes tiny, we have kept the serving sizes realistic. That is the good news. However, you must stay within the recommended portion sizes. That means no cheating. Otherwise you will be eating too many calories to allow for effective and continued weight loss.

Note: For those people who must monitor their sodium intake – and anyone who wants to cut down on the amount of salt in their diet – use low-sodium ingredients and salt substitutes wherever possible. Most of the recipes do not have any added salt; if you do add salt, be aware that the sodium level will go up considerably.

SEROTONIN SURGE LUNCHES

SAUTÉED SCALLOPS

This recipe can also be made with any thick, fresh fish cut into 2.5-cm (1-in) chunks in place of the scallops. If you make this substitution, reduce the serving size to 115 g (4 oz) for women and 170 g (6 oz) for men.

Scallops
> *Women: 170 g (6 oz)/Men: 250 g (9 oz)*

1 tablespoon flour

½ teaspoon dried basil or dried marjoram

Olive oil cooking spray

1 teaspoon olive oil

2 teaspoons lemon juice or white wine

Put the scallops in a zip-top bag with the flour and basil or marjoram. Close the bag and shake to coat the scallops.

Heat a large frying pan over medium-high heat, coat liberally with cooking spray, and add the liquid oil.

Add the scallops and cook, stirring frequently, for 2 to 3 minutes or until crisp on the outside and moist on the inside. Add the lemon juice or wine and continue to cook until all of the liquid has evaporated.

Serve immediately.

Serve with steamed mixed vegetables topped with French Dressing (see page 254).

Makes 1 serving

Per serving (women): 210 calories, 31 g protein, 7 g carbohydrates, 6 g total fat, 1 g dietary fibre, 95 mg sodium

Per serving (men): 280 calories, 46 g protein, 7 g carbohydrates, 6 g total fat, 1 g dietary fibre, 140 mg sodium

CHEESEBURGER

Yes, you can enjoy a real cheeseburger.

> **Lean minced beef formed into a 1 cm (½ in) round burger**
> *Women: 115 g (4 oz)/Men: 170 g (6 oz)*
>
> **1 low-fat cheese slice (i.e. Dairylea Light)**
>
> **2 large lettuce leaves (romaine or iceberg)**
>
> **2 large slices tomato**
>
> **1 slice red onion**
>
> **1 tablespoon tomato ketchup**
>
> **1 tablespoon mustard**
>
> **3–5 slices pickled gherkin or thin cucumber slices to reduce sodium intake (optional)**

Over high heat, grill or pan-sear the burger for 3 minutes on one side. Flip and cook until almost done, 1 additional minute. Top with the cheese and cook until the cheese melts. Build your cheeseburger between the lettuce leaves using the remaining ingredients.

Serve with Coleslaw (see page 244).

Makes 1 serving

Per serving (women): 287 calories, 30 g protein, 14 g carbohydrates, 12 g total fat, 2 g dietary fibre, 625 mg sodium

Per serving (men): 383 calories, 42 g protein, 14 g carbohydrates, 17 g total fat, 2 g dietary fibre, 666 mg sodium

Sirloin Steak with Mushrooms

Bottled barbecue sauce can be used as the marinade for this recipe if you're in a hurry.

MARINADE

1 tablespoon molasses

2 tablespoons tomato ketchup

1 teaspoon Worcestershire sauce

1 tablespoon low-sodium soy sauce

In a small bowl, combine the ingredients.

STEAK

Sirloin or rump steak
Women: 115 g (4 oz)/Men: 170 g (6 oz)

1 teaspoon olive oil

Olive oil cooking spray

230 g (8 oz) mushrooms, sliced

30 g (1 oz) chopped spring onions

Put the steak in a zip-top bag with the marinade. Seal the bag, shake to coat the steak, and refrigerate for at least 8 hours or overnight. Remove the steak and discard the used marinade.

Grill the steak on high heat, 1 to 2 minutes per side. Remove from heat and cut the steak diagonally against the grain. Cover with foil to keep it warm.

Heat the olive oil in a frying pan coated with cooking spray over medium heat and sauté the mushrooms for 3 minutes.

Put the sliced steak on a platter and top with the mushrooms and spring onions.

Serve with iceberg lettuce wedges topped with Chilli and Lime Dressing (see page 256).

Makes 1 serving

> *Per serving (women): 314 calories, 33 g protein, 28 g carbohydrates, 12 g total fat, 4 g dietary fibre, 551 mg sodium*

> *Per serving (men): 394 calories, 45 g protein, 28 g carbohydrates, 15 g total fat, 4 g dietary fibre, 582 mg sodium*

TUNA, TURKEY AND EGG SALAD

This salad is simple to put together so it's great for taking to work. Alternatively, if you're lucky enough to have a salad bar nearby get them to do it for you!

Tuna without mayonnaise
> *Women: 30 g (1 oz)/Men: 60 g (2 oz)*

Cooked turkey breast, chunks or sliced
> *Women: 60 g (2 oz)/Men: 90 g (3 oz)*

150–200 g (5½–7 oz) or more assorted vegetables plus lettuce

1 hard-boiled egg

2 tablespoons fat-free or low-fat dressing

Toss all of the ingredients together.

Makes 1 serving

> *Per serving (women): 237 calories, 32 g protein, 11 g carbohydrates, 7 g total fat, 3 g dietary fibre, 593 mg sodium*

> *Per serving (men): 311 calories, 47 g protein, 11 g carbohydrates, 8 g total fat, 3 g dietary fibre, 714 mg sodium*

Warm Salmon Salad

This dish works wonderfully as either a flavourful summer lunch or a brightly coloured meal on a dark winter day.

> 2 tablespoons unsweetened orange juice
>
> 120 ml (4 fl oz) white wine or water
>
> 5 cm (2 in) piece fresh ginger, peeled and coarsely chopped
>
> Salmon fillet, pink (defrost if frozen)
> > *Women: 115 g (4 oz)/Men: 170 g (6 oz)*
>
> 2 orange slices
>
> 45 g (1½ oz) rocket or baby spinach
>
> 1 tablespoon dried cranberries

In a deep frying pan, combine the orange juice, wine or water, and ginger. Bring the liquid to a simmer over medium heat, add the salmon and cook for 4 minutes. Turn the salmon over and place the orange slices on top of the salmon. Continue cooking for 3 minutes or until the fish is cooked through, adding more water or juice if the liquid evaporates completely.

Place the salmon on the rocket or spinach and top with the cranberries.

Makes 1 serving

Per serving (women): 338 calories, 26 g protein, 20 g carbohydrates, 9 g total fat, 4 g dietary fibre, 139 mg sodium

Per serving (men): 428 calories, 38 g protein, 20 g carbohydrates, 13 g total fat, 4 g dietary fibre, 165 mg sodium

Lemony Chicken

This dish reheats beautifully. When you make it for lunch, make extra portions for your family's dinner.

Salt (optional)

Ground black pepper

Boneless, skinless chicken breast, pounded flat
Women: 115 g (4 oz)/Men: 170 g (6 oz)

1 tablespoon flour

2 teaspoons olive oil

240 ml (8 fl oz) chicken or vegetable stock

Juice from 1 lemon

30 g (1 oz) chopped fresh Italian parsley

Lemon slices (optional)

Sprinkle salt (if desired) and pepper on the chicken to season it. Put the flour and chicken in a zip-top bag and shake to coat the chicken.

In a large frying pan, heat the oil over medium-high heat. Shake the excess flour off the chicken and place it in the pan, cooking it until golden brown on both sides (approximately 2 minutes per side). Add the stock and lemon juice to this pan and simmer for about 5 minutes or until the stock is reduced to a thick liquid. Add the parsley and cook for another 2 minutes.

Put the chicken on a plate with the thickened stock. Garnish with lemon slices if desired.

NOTE: If you're having a hard time getting juice from the lemon, try microwaving it for 10 seconds.

Serve with Lemon Garlic Spinach (see page 244).

Makes 1 serving

Per serving (women): 253 calories, 32 g protein, 8 g carbohydrates, 12 g total fat, 4 g dietary fibre, 460 mg sodium

Per serving (men): 319 calories, 45 g protein, 8 g carbohydrates, 14 g total fat, 4 g dietary fibre, 488 mg sodium

Halibut with Peppers

Prepare an extra batch of the garlic, pepper and onion mixture and use it as a topping for baked potatoes or rice.

> 2 teaspoons olive oil
>
> 2–3 cloves garlic, crushed
>
> 1 pepper, sliced (choose a yellow, red or orange pepper)
>
> 1 onion, sliced
>
> Salt (optional)
>
> Ground black pepper
>
> 240 ml (8 fl oz) low-sodium chicken or vegetable stock
>
> 4 tablespoons chopped fresh basil or 2 teaspoons dried basil
>
> Halibut fillet
> > *Women: 115 g (4 oz)/Men: 170 g (6 oz)*

Heat the oil over medium heat in a large frying pan. Add the garlic, sliced pepper and onion and sauté until tender, approximately 4 minutes. Season with salt, if desired, and pepper. Add the stock and basil. Cook 1 minute longer.

Sprinkle the fish with salt, if desired, and pepper and place on top of the pepper mixture. Cover and reduce heat.

Simmer for 7 to 8 minutes or until the fish flakes easily with a fork.

Makes 1 serving

Per serving (women): 342 calories, 32 g protein, 26 g carbohydrates, 13 g total fat, 7 g dietary fibre, 145 mg sodium

Per serving (men): 404 calories, 44 g protein, 26 g carbohydrates, 15 g total fat, 6 g dietary fibre, 175 mg sodium

SEROTONIN BALANCE AND CONTROL LUNCHES

ASIAN CHICKEN WRAP

The chicken mixture can be made ahead of time and refrigerated, which makes this recipe fast and convenient for lunch.

1 teaspoon sesame or olive oil

1 teaspoon crushed garlic

30 g (1 oz) chopped spring onions

75 g (2½ oz) grated cabbage and carrot

Boneless cooked chicken breast, sliced thin
> Women: 90 g (3 oz)/Men: 145 g (5 oz)

1½ tablespoons hoisin sauce

1 teaspoon ground black pepper

10 large lettuce leaves

Heat the oil in a large frying pan over low-medium heat. Add the garlic, spring onions, cabbage and carrots, chicken, hoisin sauce and pepper. Cook for 5 to 7 minutes, until the cabbage is soft. Remove from heat and allow to cool slightly. Spoon the mixture onto the lettuce leaves and wrap.

Serve with steamed pak choi or broccoli.

Makes 1 serving

Per serving (women): 295 calories, 29 g protein, 24 g carbohydrates, 9 g total fat, 6 g dietary fibre, 510 mg sodium

Per serving (men): 389 calories, 47 g protein, 24 g carbohydrates, 10 g total fat, 6 g dietary fibre, 552 mg sodium

Prawn and Fennel Stir-fry

This dish also tastes good cold. If you don't like fennel, substitute white mushrooms.

> 2 teaspoons olive oil
>
> 1 fennel bulb (about 200 g/7 oz), cut into thin slices
>
> 1 teaspoon ground black pepper
>
> 2 cloves garlic, crushed
>
> 1 teaspoon red chilli flakes or hot sauce
>
> Large prawns, uncooked, peeled (and deveined if necessary)
> *Women: 115 g (4 oz)/Men: 170 g (6 oz)*
>
> 2 tablespoons lime juice

Heat the oil in a large nonstick frying pan over medium heat.

Add the fennel, pepper and garlic and cook for 5 minutes or until the fennel is tender but not mushy.

Add the red chilli flakes and prawns. Cook 4 to 5 minutes, stirring occasionally, until the prawns are pink.

Add the lime juice and serve.

Makes 1 serving

Per serving (women): 296 calories, 29 g protein, 21 g carbohydrates, 12 g total fat, 7 g dietary fibre, 515 mg sodium

Per serving (men): 389 calories, 47 g protein, 21 g carbohydrates, 14 g total fat, 7 g dietary fibre, 645 mg sodium

SEARED SPICY TUNA SALAD

This recipe is great for a family get-together. It combines freshly cooked tuna with a crunchy salad. All the ingredients can be found in a large supermarket. Do not worry if you have to omit one of the spices; the dish will still taste good.

MARINADE

1 teaspoon sesame oil

1 tablespoon hoisin sauce

1 teaspoon five-spice powder

1 teaspoon chilli powder

In a small bowl, combine all the ingredients and set aside.

SEARED TUNA

Tuna steak
Women: 90 g (3 oz)/Men: 145 g (5 oz)

Olive oil cooking spray

Pour the marinade over the tuna and let it sit for 10 minutes. Drain the tuna, discarding the excess marinade.

Coat a large nonstick frying pan with cooking spray and heat over medium-high heat. Add the tuna, pan-frying for 2 to 3 minutes on each side or until the tuna is cooked through. Remove the tuna from the pan and let it cool. Cut the tuna into 2.5 cm (1 in) cubes and set aside.

DRESSING

1½ tablespoons low-sodium soy sauce

2 tablespoons rice vinegar

1 tablespoon honey

1 teaspoon sesame oil

2 teaspoons grated fresh ginger (optional)

1 tablespoon mirin (sweet rice wine)

2 tablespoons fresh coriander

In a small bowl, combine all of the ingredients and set aside.

SALAD

75 g (2½ oz) shredded Chinese cabbage and lambs lettuce

50 g (1¾ oz) grated carrots

30 g (1 oz) mangetout (cut in half if larger than 5 cm/2 in long)

2 spring onions, chopped

1 teaspoon sesame seeds

In a large bowl, combine the cabbage and lettuce, carrots, mangetout and spring onions. Toss with the dressing, top with the cooled tuna chunks and garnish with the sesame seeds.

Makes 1 serving

Per serving (women): 374 calories, 24 g protein, 41 g carbohydrates, 13 g total fat, 6 g dietary fibre, 882 mg sodium

Per serving (men): 432 calories, 36 g protein, 41 g carbohydrates, 14 g total fat, 6 g dietary fibre, 1,006 mg sodium

SWEET AND SPICY CHICKEN

This flavourful recipe tastes like it should be complicated, but it is really simple to prepare.

1 teaspoon butter

Olive oil cooking spray

Boneless, skinless chicken breast
Women: 115 g (4 oz)/Men: 170 g (6 oz)

1 teaspoon chilli powder or Caribbean jerk seasoning

1 clove garlic, crushed

80 ml (3 fl oz) orange juice

2 tablespoons lime juice

60 ml (2 fl oz) white wine

1 tablespoon sesame seeds

1 slice orange

Melt the butter in a large nonstick frying pan coated with cooking spray over medium-high heat. Sprinkle both sides of the chicken breast with chilli powder or jerk seasoning. Sear the chicken for 1 minute on each side.

Reduce the heat to medium. Add the garlic and cook for 1 minute.

Add the orange and lime juices and wine. Cook the chicken breast for an additional 2 to 3 minutes on each side, occasionally scraping the juices from the pan, until the chicken is cooked through. Sprinkle with the sesame seeds, top with the orange slice and serve.

Makes 1 serving

Per serving (women): 312 calories, 29 g protein, 17 g carbohydrates, 10 g total fat, 2 g dietary fibre, 165 mg sodium

Per serving (men): 375 calories, 42 g protein, 17 g carbohydrates, 11 g total fat, 2 g dietary fibre, 202 mg sodium

Beef Stir-Fry

This dish also works well with chicken, prawns or tofu instead of beef.
If you don't like your foods too spicy, eliminate the chilli-garlic sauce.

> 120 ml (4 fl oz) low-sodium chicken stock
>
> 1 tablespoon low-sodium soy sauce
>
> 1 tablespoon sugar-free orange marmalade or
>   sugar-free apricot jam
>
> 1½ teaspoons hoisin sauce
>
> 1 tablespoon rice vinegar
>
> 1 tablespoon cornflour
>
> 1 teaspoon bottled chilli-garlic sauce (optional)
>
> Olive oil cooking spray
>
> 1 teaspoon rapeseed oil
>
> Lean beef, thinly sliced
>   *Women: 90 g (3 oz)/Men: 145 g (5 oz)*
>
> 230 g (8 oz) frozen stir-fry vegetable mix

In a medium bowl, mix 60 ml (2 fl oz) of chicken stock, the soy sauce, marmalade, hoisin sauce, vinegar, cornflour and chilli-garlic sauce (if desired). Set aside.

Heat a large frying pan coated with cooking spray. Add the oil and when that is heated, add the beef and stir-fry over high heat until browned, about 2 minutes. Remove the beef from the frying pan. Add the vegetables and the remaining 60 ml (2 fl oz) of chicken stock to the frying pan and cook until the vegetables are soft but not mushy, about 5 minutes. Stir in the sauce and cook until the sauce becomes thick. Add the beef and cook until the beef is heated through.

Makes 1 serving

Per serving (women): 347 calories, 27 g protein, 37 g carbohydrates, 12 g total fat, 6 g dietary fibre, 945 mg sodium

Per serving (men): 435 calories, 39 g protein, 37 g carbohydrates, 16 g total fat, 7 g dietary fibre, 976 mg sodium

CRUSTY TRUSTY TROUT

Fresh rainbow trout fillets are widely available and are both delicious and economical.

> Olive oil cooking spray
>
> Fresh trout fillets
> > *Women: 90 g (3 oz)/Men: 145 g (5 oz)*
>
> ¼ teaspoon ground black pepper
>
> 2 teaspoons honey mustard
>
> 30 g (1 oz) breadcrumbs (fresh or packaged)
>
> Lemon wedges

Preheat oven to 230°C/450°F/gas 8.

Line a baking tray with aluminium foil. Coat the foil with cooking spray. Place the trout, skin side down, on the foil. Season the trout with pepper. Spread the mustard on the trout and sprinkle with the breadcrumbs.

Bake for 5 minutes or until the fish flakes easily with a fork.

Serve with lemon wedges.

Serve with 150–200 g (5½–7 oz) of steamed courgette and butternut squash drizzled with fresh lemon juice and chopped fresh basil.

Makes 1 serving

Per serving (women): 287 calories, 28 g protein, 25 g carbohydrates, 6 g total fat, 0 g dietary fibre, 323 mg sodium

Per serving (men): 343 calories, 40 g protein, 25 g carbohydrates, 9 g total fat, 0 g dietary fibre, 342 mg sodium

Fish with Barbecue Sauce

This recipe makes enough sauce to use later on chicken, beef or pork. The sauce keeps for a week in the refrigerator. The fish, which can be barbecued or grilled, can also be eaten cold the day after cooking.

SAUCE

2 tablespoons orange juice

1 tablespoon sugar-free apricot jam

2 tablespoons lime juice

½ teaspoon finely chopped fresh ginger (optional)

½ teaspoon Dijon or other strong mustard

¼ teaspoon nutmeg

¼ teaspoon allspice or cinnamon

Combine all of the ingredients in a saucepan over high heat. Bring to the boil. Lower the heat and simmer for 5 minutes.

FISH

Ground black pepper

Firm, white fish, like halibut
Women: 90 g (3 oz)/Men: 145 g (5 oz)

Olive oil cooking spray

Sprinkle the pepper on the fish to season it and place the fish on a barbecue grill rack heated over high heat or on a grill pan heated on high heat and coated with cooking spray. Cook on one side for 4 minutes. Turn the fish and brush with the sauce. Cook on the other side for 3 minutes or until the fish flakes easily. Brush with sauce and serve.

Makes 1 serving

Per serving (women): 239 calories, 36 g protein, 13 g carbohydrates, 4 g total fat, 0 g dietary fibre, 126 mg sodium

Per serving (men): 301 calories, 48 g protein, 13 g carbohydrates, 5 g total fat, 0 g dietary fibre, 156 mg sodium

Roast Chicken and Vegetables

It seems that everyone has a favourite roast chicken recipe. This is one of ours.

>Olive oil cooking spray
>
>Skinless chicken breast
>>*Women: 90 g (3 oz)/Men: 145 g (5 oz)*
>
>½ large red onion, cut into 2.5 cm (1 in) chunks
>
>1 small courgette, cut into 2.5 cm (1 in) chunks
>
>2 celery sticks, cut into 2.5 cm (1 in) chunks
>
>1 small carrot, cut into 2.5 cm (1 in) chunks
>
>1 teaspoon olive oil
>
>2 tablespoons balsamic vinegar
>
>1 teaspoon garlic granules
>
>½ teaspoon dried thyme
>
>½ teaspoon dried basil
>
>½ teaspoon dried oregano
>
>Ground black pepper

Preheat the oven to 200°C/400°F/gas 6. Coat the bottom of a deep roasting tin with cooking spray.

Place the chicken breast in the pan. Add the vegetables, olive oil and vinegar. Toss well to coat the chicken and vegetables. Spray lightly with cooking spray. Sprinkle with the garlic granules, herbs and pepper and toss again. Roast for 45 minutes, removing the pan from the oven every 15 minutes to stir the contents to ensure even cooking.

Makes 1 serving

Per serving (women): 245 calories, 24 g protein, 26 g carbohydrates, 6 g total fat, 7 g dietary fibre, 197 mg sodium

Per serving (men): 308 calories, 37 g protein, 26 g carbohydrates, 7 g total fat, 7 g dietary fibre, 234 mg sodium

TUNA CHOPPED SALAD

Marinating the onion in this recipe gives it a smoother flavour, but you can skip this step if you don't have time. To make preparing this recipe even quicker, use leftover steamed vegetables such as green beans, cauliflower, asparagus and broccoli.

> 1 small red onion, thinly sliced
>
> 2 tablespoons red vinegar or balsamic vinegar
>
> 150–200 g (5½–7 oz) mixture of any of the following vegetables, cooked or raw:
>
> Green beans, chopped
>
> Carrots, sliced or grated
>
> Cherry tomatoes
>
> Cauliflower florets
>
> Broccoli florets
>
> Radishes, sliced
>
> Asparagus, chopped
>
> Cucumber, chopped
>
> Tuna, canned in oil, well drained
> > *Women: 90 g (3 oz)/Men: 145 g (5 oz)*
>
> Ground black pepper

Marinate the onion in the vinegar for 30 minutes or longer.

Combine the onion with the remaining ingredients. Add pepper to taste and serve on a bed of lettuce.

Makes 1 serving

Per serving (women): 319 calories, 35 g protein, 25 g carbohydrates, 10 g total fat, 7 g dietary fibre, 341 mg sodium

Per serving (men): 425 calories, 50 g protein, 25 g carbohydrates, 14 g total fat, 7 g dietary fibre, 369 mg sodium

SEROTONIN SURGE DINNERS

In these recipes, you'll see that many of the carbohydrates are combined with others. Beans can be added to a rice salad, or a vegetable dish can be wrapped in a tortilla. Corn on the cob, crusty bread and a gazpacho soup may be a summer dinner. Feel free to create your own combinations of carbohydrates, using the following recipes as a starting point.

PAD THAI SALAD

For an interesting change, try this easy version of a Thai classic.

> 60 ml (2 fl oz) rice vinegar
>
> 1 tablespoon low-sodium soy sauce
>
> 1 tablespoon sugar
>
> ½ teaspoon crushed garlic
>
> Dash of sesame oil
>
> Chinese noodles (rice, stir-fry or wheat), cooked according to package directions and cooled
> > *Women: 230 g (8 oz)/Men: 320 g (11 oz)*
>
> 75 g (2½ oz) grated carrot
>
> 4 tablespoons chopped fresh coriander
>
> 1 teaspoon chopped peanuts (optional)
>
> 45 g (1½ oz) baby spinach

In a large bowl, combine the vinegar, soy sauce, sugar, garlic and sesame oil.

Add the noodles, carrot and coriander. Toss to combine. Stir in the peanuts, if desired, and serve over the spinach.

Makes 1 serving

Per serving (women): 441 calories, 7 g protein, 92 g carbohydrates, 5 g total fat, 8 g dietary fibre, 712 mg sodium

Per serving (men): 537 calories, 8 g protein, 114 g carbohydrates, 5 g total fat, 9 g dietary fibre, 726 mg sodium

Italian Flag Salad

If you have time, make this as much as a day ahead so that the flavours can blend.

> **285 g (10 oz) fresh baby spinach leaves or frozen chopped spinach**
>
> **1 tablespoon olive oil**
>
> **1 small red onion, chopped**
>
> **Canned cannellini or small white beans, well rinsed and drained**
> *Women: 375 g (13 oz)/Men: 500 g (1 lb 2 oz)*
>
> **150 g (5½ oz) cherry tomatoes**
>
> **1 teaspoon Italian seasoning**
>
> **Salt (optional)**
>
> **Ground black pepper**
>
> **1 teaspoon balsamic vinegar**

Heat a large, deep nonstick frying pan over medium heat.

Add the spinach to the ungreased pan and cook for 2 to 3 minutes or until the spinach is wilted (or heated through if using frozen).

Transfer the spinach to a large bowl and set aside.

Reduce the pan heat to low-medium. Add the olive oil and onion to the pan and sauté for 3 minutes or until the onion is soft.

Add the beans and heat through, approximately 2 minutes.

Add the bean mixture, tomatoes, seasoning, salt (if desired), pepper and vinegar to the spinach and mix well.

Makes 1 serving

Per serving (women): 429 calories, 31 g protein, 81 g carbohydrates, 10 g total fat, 27 g dietary fibre, 300 mg sodium

Per serving (men): 509 calories, 38 g protein, 100 g carbohydrates, 11 g total fat, 33 g dietary fibre, 315 mg sodium

Mushroom Burger

This is a sandwich everyone in your family will enjoy. Give yourself enough time to marinate the mushrooms so they become very flavourful.

2 tablespoons low-sodium soy sauce

½ tablespoon olive or rapeseed oil

2 tablespoons balsamic vinegar

3 cloves garlic, crushed

2 x 10 cm (4 in) portabella mushroom caps

Crusty French bread

> *Women: 15 cm- (6-in)-long thin baguette, cut in half*
> *Men: 20 cm- (8-in)-long thin baguette, cut in half*

3 slices tomato

2 leaves romaine lettuce

2 thin slices red onion

Ketchup (optional)

Mustard (optional)

Relish (optional)

Combine the soy sauce, oil, vinegar and garlic in a zip-top bag.

Add the mushrooms, seal the bag and shake gently to coat the mushrooms. Marinate at room temperature for 2 hours, gently shaking the bag occasionally. Remove the mushrooms and discard the bag and the remaining marinade.

Preheat the oven to 260°C/500°F/highest gas setting. Place the mushrooms on a grill pan or baking tray and roast for 4 minutes. Turn the mushrooms over and cook for another 2 to 3 minutes. Remove the mushrooms and set them aside, covering them with foil to keep them warm.

To assemble the sandwich, put the mushrooms on one-half of the bread. Top with the tomato, lettuce, onion and the condiments of your choice. Top with the other half of the bread.

Serve with Oh Hot Tomato! (see page 249).

Makes 1 serving

Per serving (women): 316 calories, 12 g protein, 47 g carbohydrates, 9 g total fat, 6 g dietary fibre, 1,429 mg sodium

Per serving (men): 394 calories, 15 g protein, 62 g carbohydrates, 10 g total fat, 7 g dietary fibre, 1,601 mg sodium

Sushi Rice Salad

If you like sushi rolls, you'll love this Japanese-inspired rice dish.

2 tablespoons rice vinegar

1 teaspoon rapeseed oil

1 teaspoon sesame oil

2 teaspoons low-sodium soy sauce

1 teaspoon grated fresh ginger (optional)

Short-grain or sushi rice, cooked according to package directions
> *Women: 300 g (10½ oz)/Men: 400 g (14 oz)*

125 g (4½ oz) peeled and finely chopped cucumber

30 g (1 oz) grated carrot

½ small red onion, finely chopped

2 teaspoons sesame seeds

In a small bowl, combine the vinegar, vegetable oil, sesame oil, soy sauce, and ginger, if desired.

Put the cooked rice in a large bowl. Pour the vinegar mixture over the rice.

Add the cucumber, carrot and onion and mix well. Sprinkle with the sesame seeds before serving.

Makes 1 serving

Per serving (women): 418 calories, 8 g protein, 66 g carbohydrates, 13 g total fat, 7 g dietary fibre, 392 mg sodium

Per serving (men): 503 calories, 10 g protein, 85 g carbohydrates, 13 g total fat, 7 g dietary fibre, 397 mg sodium

FAST CREAMY BROCCOLI RICE

Two kinds of cheese give this recipe a savoury taste.

> 2 tablespoons low-sodium chicken stock or water
>
> 285 g (10 oz) frozen broccoli florets
>
> Cooked rice, white or brown, reheated according to package directions
> > *Women: 230 g (8 oz)/Men: 320 g (11 oz)*
>
> 1 low-fat or light Swiss cheese slice
>
> 1 tablespoon Parmesan cheese
>
> Ground white pepper

In a large frying pan over medium-high heat, heat the chicken stock and broccoli florets until the broccoli is thawed. Add the rice and stir to mix. Top the rice with cheeses and heat, stirring occasionally, until the cheese is melted. Season with pepper to taste.

Makes 1 serving

Per serving (women): 430 calories, 32 g protein, 71 g carbohydrates, 2 g total fat, 10 g dietary fibre, 562 mg sodium

Per serving (men): 512 calories, 34 g protein, 90 g carbohydrates, 3 g total fat, 10 g dietary fibre, 565 mg sodium

Spaghetti with Roasted Courgette and Onion

You can use other roasted vegetables, such as asparagus, brussels sprouts or peppers, in this recipe.

> **Olive oil cooking spray**
>
> **1 medium courgette, thickly sliced**
>
> **½ medium onion, thickly sliced**
>
> **½ teaspoon ground black pepper**
>
> **Spaghetti, cooked according to package directions**
> *Women: 200 g (7 oz)/Men: 285 g (10 oz)*
>
> **1½ tablespoons Parmesan cheese**

Preheat oven to 260°C/500°F/highest gas setting. Line two large baking trays with aluminium foil and coat with cooking spray.

Put the courgette and onions on the trays, sprinkle with the pepper and coat lightly with cooking spray.

Roast for 8 to 10 minutes or until the vegetables are tender inside but crisp on the outside.

Add the vegetables to the cooked pasta and toss to mix. Top the pasta with the Parmesan cheese.

Serve with a mixed green salad tossed with Italian Dressing (see page 255).

Makes 1 serving

Per serving (women): 383 calories, 16 g protein, 74 g carbohydrates, 2 g total fat, 8 g dietary fibre, 115 mg sodium

Per serving (men): 481 calories, 19 g protein, 94 g carbohydrates, 2 g total fat, 8 g dietary fibre, 156 mg sodium

Indian Roasted Potato Chunks with Mint and Yogurt Dipping Sauce

The hot spiciness of the potato chunks is balanced by the cool mint and yogurt sauce.

DIPPING SAUCE

180 g (6½ oz) fat-free natural yogurt

1 medium cucumber, peeled and chopped or grated

2 tablespoons chopped fresh mint

1 tablespoon low-sugar marmalade

¼ teaspoon cayenne pepper or hot sauce

Ground black pepper

Combine all the ingredients in a small bowl.

POTATOES

2 teaspoons rapeseed oil

2 tablespoons curry powder

Ground black pepper

Baking potatoes, cut into chunks
> *Women: 230 g (8 oz)/Men: 310 g (11 oz)*

Olive oil cooking spray

Preheat the oven to 230°C/450°F/gas 8.

Put the olive oil, curry powder, pepper and potato chunks in a zip-top bag. Close the bag and shake to coat the potatoes.

Coat a baking tray with cooking spray and place the potatoes on the baking tray.

Bake for I hour or until the potatoes are well browned and crisp.

Serve hot or at room temperature with dipping sauce.

Serve with steamed vegetables, such as green beans or broccoli.

Makes 1 serving

Per serving (women): 412 calories, 10 g protein, 71 g carbohydrates, 11 g total fat, 12 g dietary fibre, 189 mg sodium

Per serving (men): 471 calories, 12 g protein, 85 g carbohydrates, 11 g total fat, 14 g dietary fibre, 194 mg sodium

TABOULI

This salad can be put together quickly with brown rice if you have some on hand. Just use it in place of the bulgur. The amounts of vegetables in this dish do not have to be precise, so you can use whatever you have in the refrigerator. This is also a great salad to take to a barbecue.

Bulgur (cracked wheat), prepared according to package directions and cooled
   Women: 180 g (6½ oz)/Men: 275 g (9¼ oz)

90 g (3 oz) chopped tomatoes or halved cherry tomatoes

¼ cucumber, peeled and chopped

¼ red onion, finely chopped, or spring onions, chopped

1 red, yellow or orange pepper, finely chopped

1 tablespoon sliced black olives (optional)

2 teaspoons olive oil

1 tablespoon crumbled feta cheese

1 tablespoon balsamic vinegar

30 g (1 oz) chopped fresh parsley

Ground black pepper

Lettuce leaves

In a large bowl, combine all of the ingredients. Serve on lettuce leaves or use them as wraps for the tabouli.

Makes 1 serving

Per serving (women): 342 calories, 11 g protein, 53 g carbohydrates, 12 g total fat, 15 g dietary fibre, 160 mg sodium

Per serving (men): 418 calories, 14 g protein, 69 g carbohydrates, 13 g total fat, 17 g dietary fibre, 165 mg sodium

Potato Pancakes

If you use the grating disc on a food processor, this recipe takes only minutes to prepare.

> Grated baking potatoes
>> *Women: 285 g (10 oz)/Men: 340 g (12 oz)*
>
> 1 tablespoon flour
>
> ¼ teaspoon ground black pepper
>
> 1 egg white
>
> Olive oil cooking spray
>
> 1 teaspoon rapeseed oil
>
> 60 g (2 oz) unsweetened apple sauce
>
> 3 tablespoons fat-free or low-fat soured cream or crème fraîche

In a large bowl, combine the potatoes, flour and pepper.

Add the egg white and mix until combined.

Coat a large nonstick frying pan with cooking spray and heat the oil over medium heat.

Drop the potato mixture in the oil in 60 ml (2 fl oz) measurements, keeping each pancake from touching.

Cook about 3 minutes on each side or until browned. Remove the pancakes from the pan and drain on kitchen towels. Repeat with the remaining mixture.

Top with apple sauce and soured cream.

Makes 1 serving

Per serving (women): 368 calories, 12 g protein, 70 g carbohydrates, 5 g total fat, 7 g dietary fibre, 142 mg sodium

Per serving (men): 412 calories, 13 g protein, 80 g carbohydrates, 5 g total fat, 9 g dietary fibre, 145 mg sodium

RED LENTIL AND CAULIFLOWER CURRY

Though this recipe has quite a few ingredients, several are spices that can be added very quickly. Best of all, you don't have to stay in the kitchen while the lentils cook.

Olive oil cooking spray

½ tablespoon rapeseed or vegetable oil

½ small onion, chopped

2 cloves garlic, crushed

Dried (uncooked) red lentils, rinsed
Women: 60 g (2 oz)/Men: 90 g (3 oz)

480 ml (16 fl oz) water or low-sodium chicken or vegetable stock

400 g can chopped tomatoes

125 g (4½ oz) frozen cauliflower florets

1 teaspoon cumin

1 teaspoon curry powder (preferably Madras)

¼ teaspoon cayenne pepper

Coat a large saucepan with cooking spray over medium heat. Add the oil and cook the onion and garlic until they are fragrant, about 2 minutes. Add the lentils and water or stock and bring to a simmer. Cover and cook for about 45 minutes or until the lentils are soft, adding more liquid if the saucepan contents become dry.

Add the tomatoes, cauliflower, cumin, curry powder and cayenne pepper and cook for 10 minutes.

Makes 1 serving

Per serving (women): 412 calories, 23 g protein, 65 g carbohydrates, 10 g total fat, 18 g dietary fibre, 592 mg sodium

Per serving (men): 548 calories, 34 g protein, 87 g carbohydrates, 11 g total fat, 23 g dietary fibre, 596 mg sodium

Buckwheat with Farfalle Pasta

This recipe is an excellent example of carb-combining.

> **Buckwheat, cooked according to package directions**
> *Women: 125 g (4½ oz)/Men: 170 g (6 oz)*
>
> **Farfalle pasta, cooked according to package directions**
> *Women: 100 g (3½ oz)/Men: 145 g (5 oz)*
>
> **1 tablespoon melted butter**
>
> **Salt (optional)**
>
> **Ground black pepper (optional)**

Combine the cooked buckwheat and the cooked pasta. Add the butter, then salt and pepper to taste if desired. Mix to combine.

Serve with a mixed greens and tomato salad topped with a dressing of your choice (see pages 254–57).

Makes 1 serving

Per serving (women): 362 calories, 9 g protein, 51 g carbohydrates, 15 g total fat, 5 g dietary fibre, 293 mg sodium

Per serving (men): 441 calories, 11 g protein, 68 g carbohydrates, 15 g total fat, 7 g dietary fibre, 295 mg sodium

TIP: Experiment with different starches now commonly found in health food shops. Among these is buckwheat. Buckwheat is actually a berry, not a grain, and it is high in fibre and has a nutty flavour. Also try millet and quinoa, which are high-fibre, nutritious grains. Buckwheat, millet and quinoa can be boiled in water or stock, using 2 parts liquid for every 1 part starch.

SEROTONIN BALANCE AND CONTROL DINNERS

ASIAN RICE AND PRAWN SALAD

Chicken or tofu can be substituted for the prawns in this recipe.

Jasmine or medium-grain rice, cooked according to package directions
> *Women: 285 g (10 oz)/Men: 375 g (13 oz)*

Cooked prawns, warm or cool
> *Women: 60 g (2 oz)/Men: 90 g (3 oz)*

60 ml (2 fl oz) fat-free or reduced-fat coconut milk

2 teaspoons rice vinegar

1 teaspoon rapeseed oil

3 tablespoons chopped fresh basil

½ tablespoon chopped salted peanuts

Combine the rice and cooked prawns in a bowl. In a separate bowl, combine the coconut milk, vinegar, oil and basil and then add it to the rice and prawn mixture. Toss to combine and sprinkle with chopped peanuts before serving.

Serve with steamed pak choi or Chinese cabbage topped with teriyaki or soy sauce.

Makes 1 serving

Per serving (women): 535 calories, 22 g protein, 82 g carbohydrates, 12 g total fat, 2 g dietary fibre, 223 mg sodium

Per serving (men): 725 calories, 38 g protein, 109 g carbohydrates, 13 g total fat, 2 g dietary fibre, 292 mg sodium

CRUSTY BREAD SALAD WITH CHICKEN

This is our version of panzanella, or Tuscan bread salad. It solves the problem of what to do with leftover bread.

VINAIGRETTE

1 tablespoon balsamic vinegar

2 teaspoons olive oil

½ teaspoon dried basil

½ teaspoon dried tarragon

½ teaspoon dried thyme

Ground black pepper

1 tablespoon anchovy paste (optional)

Combine all ingredients in a small bowl and set aside.

SALAD

Olive oil cooking spray

1 pepper (red, yellow or orange), cut into 2.5-cm (1-in) wide
    strips

1 yellow courgette, cut into 2 cm (¾ in) rounds

¼ medium red onion, thinly sliced

Crusty round Italian or French bread cut into 2.5 cm (1 in)
    chunks
    Women: 50 g (1¾ oz)/Men: 65 g (2¼ oz)

1 large or 2 medium tomatoes, cut into 2.5 cm (1 in) chunks

Chicken breast, grilled, warm or at room temperature, cut into
    2.5 cm (1 in) chunks
    Women: 60 g (2 oz)/Men: 115 g (4 oz)

Preheat the oven to 260°C/500°F/highest gas setting. Coat a roasting tin with cooking spray and place the pepper, courgette, onion and bread in the tin. Coat with cooking spray.

Roast until the vegetables are tender and the bread is crisp. Remove from the oven and let stand until cool.

Place vegetable and bread mixture in a bowl. Add tomatoes, chicken and vinaigrette. Toss well.

Makes 1 serving

Per serving (women): 434 calories, 28 g protein, 52 g carbohydrates, 14 g total fat, 9 g dietary fibre, 255 mg sodium

Per serving (men): 508 calories, 48 g protein, 67 g carbohydrates, 17 g total fat, 10 g dietary fibre, 302 mg sodium

Pasta Shells with Smoked Salmon

This recipe creates a sophisticated dish worthy of guests.

> Small pasta shells or orecchiette (ear-shaped pasta), cooked according to package directions
> > *Women: 200 g (7 oz)/Men: 285 g (10 oz)*
>
> ½ tablespoon butter
>
> 75 g (2½ oz) thinly sliced Savoy or green cabbage
>
> 60 ml (2 fl oz) water or chicken or vegetable stock
>
> 75 g (2½ oz) frozen peas
>
> Chopped smoked salmon (for lower sodium, use cooked salmon)
> > *Women: 60 g (2 oz)/Men: 90 g (3 oz)*
>
> 2 tablespoons fat-free or low-fat soured cream or crème fraîche
>
> Salt (optional)
>
> Ground black pepper
>
> 2 tablespoons snipped fresh dill

Put the cooked pasta in a large bowl.

Heat the butter in a nonstick frying pan over medium heat. Add the cabbage and sauté until soft, about 6 minutes. Add water or stock and bring to a simmer. Turn off the heat and add the peas. Stir the mixture into the pasta.

Add the salmon and soured cream or crème fraîche, then salt (if desired) and pepper to taste. Sprinkle with dill just before serving.

Makes 1 serving

With smoked salmon

Per serving (women): 456 calories, 25 g protein, 68 g carbohydrates, 10 g total fat, 10 g dietary fibre, 1,275 mg sodium

Per serving (men): 604 calories, 38 g protein, 84 g carbohydrates, 13 g total fat, 8 g dietary fibre, 2,409 mg sodium

With fresh salmon

Per serving (women): 491 calories, 28 g protein, 68 g carbohydrates, 12 g total fat, 8 g dietary fibre, 170 mg sodium

Per serving (men): 672 calories, 44 g protein, 84 g carbohydrates, 17 g total fat, 8 g dietary fibre, 200 mg sodium

Chicken Soup in a Hurry

Here is a quick-to-prepare Italian version of chicken soup.

480 ml (16 fl oz) low-sodium chicken stock

45 g (1½ oz) rinsed and shredded escarole, Swiss chard or
   spinach

Rice or noodles, cooked according to package directions
   Women: 230 g (8 oz)/Men: 310 g (11 oz)

Cooked chicken breast, chopped
   Women: 60 g (2 oz)/Men: 90 g (3 oz)

1½ teaspoons lemon juice

Ground white pepper

In a large pot, bring the stock to a simmer over medium heat. Add the escarole and cook for 2 minutes or until wilted.

Add the cooked rice or noodles, chicken and lemon juice, and pepper to taste.

Pour into a serving bowl.

Makes 1 serving

Per serving (women): 473 calories, 25 g protein, 81 g carbohydrates, 6 g total fat, 3 g dietary fibre, 209 mg sodium

Per serving (men): 669 calories, 43 g protein, 104 g carbohydrates, 10 g total fat, 4 g dietary fibre, 253 mg sodium

TIP: Low-fat canned or fresh soups, like asparagus, carrot and lentil, French onion, consomme, chicken or tomato, provide the base for a great dinner. Add the protein you are planning to eat as well as a variety of vegetables, such as sweetcorn, chopped tomatoes, peas or frozen mixed vegetables. Add your favourite seasoning to the soup and even a splash of sherry (the alcohol evaporates with heating, but the flavour remains).

Polenta with Mushrooms and Meat

This hearty dish is wonderful cold weather comfort food.

> Olive oil cooking spray
>
> 2 teaspoons olive oil
>
> 3 cloves garlic, crushed
>
> 115 g (4 oz) mixture roughly chopped portabella, shiitake and oyster mushrooms (or use closed cap button mushrooms)
>
> Minced lean turkey, chicken or beef
> *Women: 60 g (2 oz)/Men: 115 g (4 oz)*
>
> Polenta, cooked according to package directions or by using the recipe for Basic Polenta on page 189
> *Women: 300 g (10½ oz)/Men: 400 g (14 oz)*
>
> 1 tablespoon grated low-fat Parmesan cheese or grated reduced-fat mozzarella

Coat a frying pan with cooking spray, add the oil and heat over low-medium heat. Sauté the garlic and mushrooms in the oil until the garlic is soft and the mushrooms are cooked, about 4 minutes. Add the turkey, chicken or beef and cook until browned, about 5 minutes.

Place the polenta in a bowl and top with the mushroom mixture. Sprinkle with the cheese.

NOTE: If you'd rather not cook the polenta, buy it ready made from the supermarket. Slice the polenta into 2.5 cm (1 in) pieces and cook over medium heat in a cooking-spray-coated frying pan for 2 minutes on each side.

Serve with some steamed broccoli topped with Italian Dressing (see page 255).

Makes 1 serving

Per serving (women): 441 calories, 21 g protein, 57 g carbohydrates, 15 g total fat, 7 g dietary fibre, 163 mg sodium

Per serving (men): 590 calories, 33 g protein, 71 g carbohydrates, 17 g total fat, 9 g dietary fibre, 169 mg sodium

CAJUN PRAWN STEW

Traditionally this dish is made to feed a crowd – if you wish to do this just increase the proportions accordingly.

2 litres (3½ pt) water

2 lemons, halved

2 teaspoons cayenne pepper

2 bay leaves

3 tablespoons seafood spice mix (or use a mixture of
   1 teaspoon dry mustard, 2 teaspoons coriander seeds,
   1 teaspoon allspice, ½ teaspoon ground cloves,
   4 bay leaves and 1 teaspoon red chilli flakes)

4 cloves garlic, peeled

1 large onion, peeled and left whole

New potatoes
   Women: 170 g (6 oz)/Men: 230 g (8 oz)

Corn on the cob
   Women: ½/Men: 1

Prawns
   Women: 30 g (1 oz)/Men: 60 g (2 oz)

Low-fat chicken, beef or pork sausage, sliced
   Women: 30 g (1 oz)/Men: 60 g (2 oz)

Bring the water to the boil in a large pot over high heat and reduce to medium-high. Squeeze the lemon juice into the water and drop the halves into the pot. Add the cayenne pepper, bay leaves, spice mix and garlic and boil for 3 minutes. Add the onion and boil for 3 minutes. Add the potatoes and cook for 3 minutes. Add the corn, prawns and sausage and boil for an additional 3 to 4 minutes until the prawns are pink. Drain in a colander and remove the bay leaves. Top with additional seasoning and serve.

Makes 1 serving

Per serving (women): 367 calories, 17 g protein, 77 g carbohydrates, 3 g total fat, 13 g dietary fibre, 290 mg sodium

Per serving (men): 526 calories, 28 g protein; 104 g carbohydrates, 5 g total fat, 16 g dietary fibre, 563 mg sodium

Pasta with Meat and Mushroom-Tomato Ragu

This is a simple and delicious dish made with a mushroom sauté. The pasta and mushrooms take about the same time to cook, so the dish should be ready 12 minutes after the water boils for the pasta.

> Penne or any short pasta, cooked according to package directions
> > *Women: 145 g (5 oz)/Men: 210 g (7½ oz)*
>
> Olive oil cooking spray
>
> 1 teaspoon olive oil
>
> 2 cloves garlic, crushed
>
> 230 g (8 oz) mushrooms
>
> Lean minced beef or turkey
> > *Women: 60 g (2 oz)/Men: 115 g (4 oz)*
>
> ¼ teaspoon ground black pepper
>
> 1 teaspoon sugar
>
> 1 teaspoon dried Italian seasoning or several fresh basil leaves
>
> 240 ml (8 fl oz) low-sodium reduced-fat or fat-free jarred tomato sauce or passata
>
> 1 tablespoon grated light mozzarella cheese

Place drained pasta back into the pot. Set aside. Coat a large frying pan with cooking spray, add the oil and warm over medium-high heat. Sauté the garlic, mushrooms and minced beef or turkey for 5 minutes or until the mushrooms are soft. Add the pepper, sugar and Italian seasoning or basil and continue cooking for 2 to 3 minutes, stirring several times. Add the mushroom mixture and tomato sauce or passata to the pasta and heat until warm. Put in a large bowl and sprinkle with the cheese.

Serve with Lemon Garlic Spinach (see page 244).

Makes 1 serving

Per serving (women): 473 calories, 30 g protein, 65 g carbohydrates, 13 g total fat, 8 g dietary fibre, 772 mg sodium

Per serving (men): 649 calories, 44 g protein, 81 g carbohydrates, 19 g total fat, 9 g dietary fibre, 814 mg sodium

Curried Thai Sweet Potato and Chicken Soup

This spicy, satisfying soup is easy to make.

> **Sweet potatoes, peeled and cut into 1 cm (½ in) chunks**
> *Women: 230 g (8 oz)/Men: 340 g (12 oz)*
>
> **480 ml (16 fl oz) low-sodium chicken or vegetable stock**
>
> **1 teaspoon rapeseed or vegetable oil**
>
> **½ medium onion, chopped**
>
> **2.5 cm (1 in) piece fresh ginger, peeled and minced (optional)**
>
> **2 teaspoons Thai curry powder**
>
> **4 tablespoons canned fat-free or reduced-fat coconut milk**
>
> **2 tablespoons lemon juice**
>
> **Cooked chicken breast, shredded**
> *Women: 60 g (2 oz)/Men: 115 g (4 oz)*
>
> **Ground black pepper**
>
> **Fresh coriander to taste**

In a large pot over medium heat, simmer the sweet potatoes in the stock for 15 minutes until tender.

Heat the oil in a frying pan over medium heat and sauté the onion and ginger until soft, about 4 minutes. Stir in the curry powder.

Add the curry–onion mixture to the sweet potatoes and stock.

Add the coconut milk, lemon juice and chicken and heat until the soup is just about to boil, approximately 2 minutes. Season with pepper to taste.

Pour the soup into a bowl and garnish with coriander.

Serve with steamed spinach.

Makes 1 serving

Per serving (women): 435 calories, 20 g protein, 76 g carbohydrates, 6 g total fat, 10 g dietary fibre, 259 mg sodium

Per serving (men): 699 calories, 52 g protein, 104 g carbohydrates, 8 g total fat, 14 g dietary fibre, 370 mg sodium

Spicy Caribbean Potato Chunks with Steak or Pork

The interesting assortment of spices in jerk seasoning turns a plain potato into something special.

> **Baking potato, scrubbed and cut into 2.5 cm (1 in) chunks**
> *Women: 340 g (12 oz)/Men: 455 g (1 lb)*
>
> **Olive oil cooking spray**
>
> **1 teaspoon Caribbean jerk seasoning**
>
> **½ teaspoon curry powder**
>
> **½ teaspoon cumin**
>
> **½ teaspoon garlic granules**
>
> **¼ teaspoon allspice (optional)**
>
> **Beef sirloin steak or pork fillet**
> *Women: 60 g (2 oz)/Men: 115 g (4 oz)*

Preheat the oven to 230°C/450°F/gas 8. Put the potato chunks in a large mixing bowl and coat them with cooking spray. Toss the potatoes and spray them again.

In a small bowl, stir together the jerk seasoning, curry powder, cumin, garlic granules, and allspice (if desired). Sprinkle the seasoning mixture over the potatoes and mix well.

Place the seasoned potatoes in a shallow baking tray.

Bake the potatoes for 30 minutes, stirring occasionally, until tender. Remove from the oven and cover with foil to keep warm.

Heat the grill. Spray the grill rack with cooking spray and grill for 3 to 4 minutes per side until the meat is cooked through.

Serve with steamed asparagus or broccoli.

Makes 1 serving

Per serving (women): 368 calories, 18 g protein, 56 g carbohydrates, 8 g total fat, 10 g dietary fibre, 340 mg sodium

Per serving (men): 563 calories, 34 g protein, 23 g carbohydrates, 16 g total fat, 13 g dietary fibre, 383 mg sodium

CORN BURRITOS

This satisfying meal is loaded with taste, crunch, spice and colour.

Canned black beans, drained and rinsed well
Women: 90 g (3 oz)/Men: 125 g (4½ oz)

Rice, brown or white, cooked according to package directions
Women: 100 g (3½ oz)/Men: 145 g (5 oz)

1 tablespoon fresh coriander (optional)

1 tablespoon fresh lime juice (optional)

Corn tortillas (15 cm/6 in each, fat-free)
Women: 2 tortillas/Men: 4 tortillas

75 g (2½ oz) shredded lettuce

**1–3 tablespoons jarred chilli peppers, finely chopped (optional)
(wear plastic gloves when handling)**

120 ml (4 fl oz) mild or hot salsa

1 tablespoon grated reduced-fat Cheddar cheese

1 teaspoon hot sauce

**1 tablespoon fat-free or reduced-fat soured cream or crème
fraîche**

In a large bowl, mix the beans and rice together. Add the coriander and lime juice if desired.

Divide the rice and bean mixture between each tortilla. Top with the lettuce, chilli peppers, salsa, cheese and hot sauce. Fold the tortilla and microwave on high for 30 seconds to warm through.

Top with the soured cream or crème fraîche.

Makes 1 serving

Per serving (women): 385 calories, 14 g protein, 84 g carbohydrates, 5 g total fat, 15 g dietary fibre, 901 mg sodium

Per serving (men): 565 calories, 20 g protein, 114 g carbohydrates, 7 g total fat, 15 g dietary fibre, 990 mg sodium

Nam Chinese Noodles with Tofu or Chicken

This recipe is very adaptable – if you don't have any Chinese noodles you can use spaghetti.

Chinese noodles or spaghetti, cooked according to package directions
> *Women: 145 g (5 oz)/Men: 220 g (7½ oz)*

Olive oil cooking spray

1 teaspoon sesame oil

2.5 cm (1 in) piece fresh ginger, peeled and chopped

2 cloves garlic, crushed

2 tablespoons low-sodium teriyaki sauce

120 ml (4 fl oz) low-sodium chicken stock

½ tablespoon cornflour

90 g (3 oz) canned straw mushrooms or closed cup mushrooms, drained

30 g (1 oz) canned water chestnuts, drained and chopped

60 g (2 oz) mangetout or asparagus

Finely chopped firm tofu or cooked chicken breast
> *Women: 60 g (2 oz)/Men: 115 g (4 oz)*

Put the cooked noodles in a large bowl and set aside.

In a large saucepan coated with cooking spray, heat the sesame oil over low heat. Add the ginger and garlic and cook for 3 minutes.

Add the teriyaki sauce and 60 ml (2 fl oz) of the chicken stock and cook over medium heat for 5 minutes. In a small bowl, mix the remaining chicken stock with the cornflour until the cornflour dissolves.

Add the cornflour mixture to the teriyaki mixture and simmer for 3 minutes, until the sauce thickens. Add the mushrooms, water chestnuts, mangetout or asparagus, and tofu or chicken to the sauce and cook until heated, about 3 minutes.

Toss the cooked, drained noodles with the sauce.

Serve with chopped romaine or iceberg lettuce topped with the dressing of your choice (see page 254–57).

Makes 1 serving

With tofu

Per serving (women): 466 calories, 24 g protein, 68 g carbohydrates, 12 g total fat, 9 g dietary fibre, 923 mg sodium

Per serving (men): 647 calories, 37 g protein, 90 g carbohydrates, 18 g total fat, 12 g dietary fibre, 931 mg sodium

With chicken

Per serving (women): 477 calories, 33 g protein, 64 g carbohydrates, 9 g total fat, 8 g dietary fibre, 957 mg sodium

Per serving (men): 669 calories, 54 g protein, 85 g carbohydrates, 12 g total fat, 9 g dietary fibre, 1,000 mg sodium

Couscous with Lamb

Couscous is made from semolina wheat flour mixed with water and salt and then rolled into tiny balls that expand when combined with hot water. The dried fruit in this dish gives it a distinctive texture.

Couscous, cooked according to package directions
   Women: 150 g (5½ oz)/Men: 230 g (8 oz)

30 g (1 oz) sultanas or dried cranberries

¼ teaspoon nutmeg

Lamb chop
   Women: 60 g (2 oz)/Men: 115 g (4 oz)

Olive oil cooking spray

Preheat the oven to 230°C/450°F/gas 8. In a large bowl, combine the couscous, raisins or dried cranberries and nutmeg. Set aside. Cook the lamb for 3 minutes on a baking tray coated with cooking spray. Reduce the heat to 180°C/350°F/gas 4 and cook for an additional 5 to 7 minutes or until the desired level of doneness is reached. Serve the lamb on top of the couscous.

Serve with Sesame Mangetout (see page 251).

Makes 1 serving

Per serving (women): 426 calories, 17 g protein, 68 g carbohydrates, 9 g total fat, 5 g dietary fibre, 152 mg sodium

Per serving (men): 632 calories, 31 g protein, 86 g carbohydrates, 17 g total fat, 5 g dietary fibre, 189 mg sodium

MEAT, RICE AND BEANS WITH A KICK

The amount of 'kick' this recipe has depends on the type of chilli pepper you use. If you like your food very spicy use habaneros, if available, or include the seeds of standard supermarket chillies.

Olive oil cooking spray

Lean minced beef or turkey
   Women: 60 g (2 oz)/Men: 115 g (4 oz)

2 cloves garlic, crushed

1 onion, chopped

1 piece of jarred roasted red pepper, chopped

1 chilli pepper, finely chopped (wear plastic gloves when handling)

Brown or white rice, cooked according to package directions
   Women: 145 g (5 oz)/Men: 200 g (7 oz)

60 g (2 oz) canned white beans, drained

115 g (4 oz) canned chopped tomatoes

Coat a large frying pan with cooking spray and heat over medium heat. Add the beef or turkey and cook until browned, stirring frequently, for about 2 to 3 minutes. Add the garlic, onion, red pepper and chilli pepper and sauté until the vegetables are soft, about 3 minutes.

Remove from the heat and combine with the rice in a bowl. Add the beans and tomatoes and mix well. Serve warm.

Serve with a mixed green salad topped with Mexican Dressing (see page 256).

Makes 1 serving

Per serving (women): 469 calories, 24 g protein, 76 g carbohydrates, 7 g total fat, 10 g dietary fibre, 517 mg sodium

Per serving (men): 624 calories, 37 g protein, 87 g carbohydrates, 13 g total fat, 11 g dietary fibre, 555 mg sodium

FISH AND ROASTED ACORN SQUASH STUFFED WITH WILD RICE MIX

The rice can be prepared ahead of time and reheated in a microwave.

> Olive oil cooking spray
>
> ½ small (10 cm/4 in diameter) acorn or butternut squash, seeded but not peeled
>
> Firm fish such as halibut, sole or cod
> *Women: 60 g (2 oz)/Men: 115 g (4 oz)*
>
> ½ tablespoon olive oil
>
> ½ small onion, chopped
>
> ½ stick celery, chopped
>
> 400 ml (14 fl oz) low-sodium fat-free chicken or vegetable stock
>
> 120 ml (4 fl oz) water
>
> Long grain and wild rice mix, cooked according to package directions
> *Women: 75 g (2½ oz)/Men: 150 g (5½ oz)*
>
> 1 tablespoon dried cherries or dried cranberries
>
> ½ teaspoon nutmeg

Preheat the oven to 200°C/400°F/gas 6. Coat the surface of a large roasting tin or baking tray with cooking spray and place the squash on it, cut side down. Bake for 30 minutes or until the squash is soft. For the last 10 minutes of baking, place the fish on the pan.

In a nonstick pot, heat the oil over medium heat. Add the onion and celery and cook for 3 minutes until soft. Add the stock and water and bring to the boil. Stir in the rice, fruit and nutmeg and simmer for 25 minutes. Fill the squash with the rice mixture and serve along with the fish.

Makes 1 serving

Per serving (women): 398 calories, 23 g protein, 58 g carbohydrates, 10 g total fat, 6 g dietary fibre, 479 mg sodium

Per serving (men): 529 calories, 36 g protein, 77 g carbohydrates, 11 g total fat, 7 g dietary fibre, 483 mg sodium

Couscous with Courgette and Chicken

If you make this dish ahead of time, microwave it to heat it through before serving.

½ tablespoon olive oil

1 small onion, chopped

½ teaspoon cumin

½ teaspoon cinnamon

½ teaspoon curry powder

2 small courgettes, cut crosswise into 5 mm (¼ in) rounds

Cooked chicken breast, cut into 1 cm (½ in) pieces
Women: 60 g (2 oz)/Men: 115 g (4 oz)

Couscous, cooked according to package directions
Women: 115 g (4 oz)/Men: 200 g (7 oz)

60 g (2 oz) canned chickpeas, drained

1 tablespoon sultanas

Ground black pepper

In a large frying pan, heat the oil over low-medium heat. Add the onion, cumin, cinnamon and curry powder and cook for 3 to 4 minutes until the onion is soft. Add the courgette and cook until tender, about 4 minutes. Add the chicken, couscous and chickpeas and heat through. Toss the sultanas into the mixture just before serving. Season with pepper to taste.

Serve with a mixed green salad topped with Spanish Dressing (see page 257).

Makes 1 serving

Per serving (women): 499 calories, 31 g protein, 73 g carbohydrates, 11 g total fat, 12 g dietary fibre, 243 mg sodium

Per serving (men): 680 calories, 51 g protein, 91 g carbohydrates, 13 g total fat, 13 g dietary fibre, 289 mg sodium

Niçoise-Inspired Tuna and Herbed Potato Salad

If you have time, make this recipe as much as a day in advance so the flavours have time to blend.

VINAIGRETTE

1 teaspoon Dijon mustard

2 teaspoons white wine vinegar

1 teaspoon honey

2 teaspoons olive oil

2 tablespoons chopped fresh tarragon or dill

In a small bowl, whisk together the mustard, vinegar, honey and oil. Stir in the tarragon or dill and set aside.

SALAD

Mixture of small red- and white-skinned potatoes
  Women: 285 g (10 oz)/Men: 455 g (1 lb)

50 g (1¾ oz) roughly cut green beans (fresh or frozen)

¼ medium red onion, sliced very thin

75 g (2½ oz) cherry tomatoes

Canned tuna packed in water, drained
  Women: 60 g (2 oz)/Men: 115 g (4 oz)

4 tablespoons chopped parsley

Place the potatoes in a large pot. Fill the pot with enough cool tap water to cover the potatoes. Cover the pot and bring the potatoes to the boil over high heat, then reduce the heat to low-medium to maintain a gentle boil. Cook the potatoes until tender, approximately 10 minutes. Drain and cool. Halve or quarter the potatoes. Steam the green beans for 3 to 5 minutes or until tender. Set aside and cool. In a large bowl, mix the potatoes, green beans, onion, tomatoes and tuna. Pour the vinaigrette over the potato mixture. Garnish with the parsley.

Makes 1 serving

Per serving (women): 422 calories, 21 g protein, 61 g carbohydrates, 11 g total fat, 11 g dietary fibre, 310 mg sodium

Per serving (men): 613 calories, 37 g protein, 88 g carbohydrates, 15 g total fat, 13 g dietary fibre, 534 mg sodium

ROAST BEEF ROLL-UP

Cold roast beef and ready-prepared vegetables combine to make a crunchy dinner 'sandwich'. This recipe makes a lot of filling, so mound as much as you like on the tortilla and eat the rest with a fork.

45 g (1½ oz) coleslaw mix or shredded cabbage and carrots

1 spring onion, chopped

1 teaspoon sesame oil

1 teaspoon lemon juice or rice vinegar

Ground black pepper

Rice, brown or white, cooked according to package directions
Women: 100 g (3½ oz)/Men: 150 g (5½ oz)

Flour tortillas, fat-free, 20 cm (8 in)
Women: 1 tortilla/Men: 2 tortillas

Lean roast beef from deli counter, thinly sliced
Women: 60 g (2 oz)/Men: 115 g (4 oz)

In a medium bowl, combine the coleslaw mix or cabbage and carrots, spring onion, oil and lemon juice or vinegar. Add pepper to taste.

Spoon the rice and the vegetable mixture onto the tortilla. Top with the roast beef. Fold the tortilla.

Makes 1 serving

Per serving (women): 409 calories, 22 g protein, 53 g carbohydrates, 12 g total fat, 4 g dietary fibre, 387 mg sodium

Per serving (men): 651 calories, 35 g protein, 90 g carbohydrates, 16 g total fat, 6 g dietary fibre, 741 mg sodium

Turkey Lentil Stew with Greens

This dish is tasty and easy to prepare. The amounts of dried lentils given below will yield the correct cooked amounts.

1 teaspoon olive oil

Olive oil cooking spray

2 cloves garlic, chopped

½ small onion, chopped

350 ml (12 fl oz) low-sodium low-fat chicken or vegetable stock

Uncooked red or yellow lentils
   Women: 3 tablespoons/Men: 4 tablespoons

3 small red-skinned potatoes

Handful roughly chopped Swiss chard, spring greens or spinach

1 medium tomato, chopped into 1 cm (½ in) chunks

Chopped smoked turkey breast
   Women: 30 g (1 oz)/Men: 90 g (3 oz)

½ teaspoon dried thyme

½ teaspoon dried basil

Heat the oil in a large pot coated with cooking spray over low-medium heat. Sauté the garlic and onion until soft, about 4 minutes. Add the stock, lentils and potatoes. Cover and cook for 20 minutes or until the lentils and potatoes are soft. Add the chopped greens, tomato, turkey and herbs. Simmer, covered, for 10 minutes.

Makes 1 serving

Per serving (women): 479 calories, 29 g protein, 76 g carbohydrates, 9 g total fat, 13 g dietary fibre, 472 mg sodium

Per serving (men): 579 calories, 42 g protein, 84 g carbohydrates, 10 g total fat, 15 g dietary fibre, 594 mg sodium

BARLEY AND CORN SALAD WITH CHICKEN

Quick-cooking barley and frozen sweetcorn make this grain salad a fast mix. The salad can be eaten hot or cold and makes a nice change from the more traditional pasta, potato or rice salad.

Pearl barley, cooked according to package directions
Women: 150 g (5½ oz)/Men: 230 g (8 oz)

Frozen sweetcorn
Women: 75 g (2½ oz)/Men: 125 g (4½ oz)

¼ red pepper, chopped

2 spring onions, chopped

2 tablespoons shredded fresh basil leaves

2 teaspoons lemon juice

1 teaspoon olive oil

Ground black pepper

Chicken breast, grilled, cut into 2.5 cm (1 in) chunks
Women: 60 g (2 oz)/Men: 115 g (4 oz)

Put the cooked barley in a large pot and add the sweetcorn. Cover the pot and let cook for 5 minutes over low heat until the sweetcorn is heated through. Turn the grain mixture into a large bowl and add the red pepper, spring onions, basil, lemon juice and olive oil. Season with pepper to taste. Add the chicken and toss well.

Serve with steamed green beans topped with French Dressing (see page 254).

Makes 1 serving

Per serving (women): 411 calories, 25 g protein, 63 g carbohydrates, 8 g total fat, 10 g dietary fibre, 265 mg sodium

Per serving (men): 632 calories, 45 g protein, 92 g carbohydrates, 10 g total fat, 14 g dietary fibre, 282 mg sodium

Very Fast Beef and Broccoli with Rice

Use microwave-in-the-bag rice, precut broccoli florets and presliced thin steak for a quick and delicious meal.

Olive oil cooking spray

2 cloves garlic, crushed

2 spring onions, chopped

½ teaspoon cumin

½ teaspoon ground coriander

¼ teaspoon ground black pepper

Lean beef, sliced into strips
Women: 60 g (2 oz)/115 g (4 oz)

75 g (2½ oz) tomatoes, halved

100 g (3½ oz) broccoli florets

Cooked rice
Women: 150 g (5½ oz)/Men: 230 g (8 oz)

Coat a nonstick frying pan with cooking spray. Over high heat, sauté the garlic and spring onions for 1 minute. Add the cumin, coriander, pepper and beef and cook until the beef is cooked through, about 3 minutes. Add the tomatoes and broccoli. Lower the heat to medium and cook 3 minutes more.

Serve the broccoli mixture over the rice.

Makes 1 serving

Per serving (women): 338 calories, 21 g protein, 56 g carbohydrates, 3 g total fat, 5 g dietary fibre, 173 mg sodium

Per serving (men): 510 calories, 35 g protein, 77 g carbohydrates, 6 g total fat, 6 g dietary fibre, 211 mg sodium

VEGETABLES

The dishes described here – including the soups – are substantial side dishes for lunch or dinner in all phases of the diet. Even if you 'hate' vegetables, give them a try. Unless otherwise noted, each recipe provides one serving. You can certainly mix and match your vegetables, using a half portion from two different recipes.

CARROT AND CUMIN SOUP

This soup is delicious hot or cold.

> Olive oil cooking spray
>
> 1 teaspoon olive oil
>
> 2 cloves garlic, crushed
>
> 2 tablespoons chopped onion
>
> 1 leek, white part only, chopped
>
> 1 teaspoon cumin
>
> ½ teaspoon cayenne pepper
>
> 240 ml (8 fl oz) low-sodium chicken stock
>
> 1 medium carrot, coarsely chopped, or packaged small peeled carrots or 60 g (2 oz) frozen chopped carrots
>
> Ground black pepper

In a soup pot coated with cooking spray, heat the oil over low-medium heat. Add the garlic, onion and leek and cook for 3 to 5 minutes until the vegetables are soft but not browned.

Increase the heat to medium. Add the cumin, cayenne pepper and stock and heat to a simmer.

Add the carrots. Cook until the carrots are tender, about 15 minutes. Cool. Purée the vegetable mixture in a food processor, or by using a handheld blender in the pot, until smooth. Add pepper to taste.

Makes 2 servings

Per serving: 97 calories, 4 g protein, 14 g carbohydrates, 3 g total fat, 3 g dietary fibre, 70 mg sodium

COLESLAW

If you use a bag of ready-grated cabbage and carrots you can complete this recipe in no time. You can make this recipe as much as 2 days in advance; just keep it covered and refrigerated.

30 g (1 oz) shredded cabbage

30 g (1 oz) grated carrot

½ apple, cored and finely chopped

2 tablespoons fat-free or extra light mayonnaise

1 tablespoon Dijon mustard

1 teaspoon sugar

2 teaspoons lemon juice

½ teaspoon cumin

In a large bowl, mix the ingredients.

Makes 1 serving

Per serving: 79 calories, 1 g protein, 18 g carbohydrates, 1 g total fat, 3 g dietary fibre, 46 mg sodium

LEMON GARLIC SPINACH

This is our version of a classic Italian side dish.

1 teaspoon olive oil

1 clove garlic, crushed

285 g (10 oz) frozen spinach, thawed according to package directions, or use fresh spinach

½ lemon

Ground black pepper

In a deep frying pan over medium heat, warm the oil and sauté the garlic until fragrant, about 2 minutes. Add the spinach and stir until the spinach is heated through (fresh spinach should be wilted). Squeeze the lemon over the spinach. Add pepper to taste.

Makes 2 servings

Per serving: 70 calories, 6 g protein, 8 g carbohydrates, 7 g total fat, 5 g dietary fibre, 32 mg sodium

ROASTED ASPARAGUS SPEARS WITH VINAIGRETTE

This is a simple yet delicious dish.

> ½ bunch fresh, thin asparagus, trimmed
>
> 1 teaspoon olive oil
>
> 1 teaspoon balsamic or flavoured vinegar
>
> ½ teaspoon Dijon mustard
>
> Ground black pepper

Preheat the oven to 200°C/400°F/gas 6. Line a baking tray with aluminium foil. Arrange the asparagus spears on the baking tray in a single row and roast until crisp on the outside but tender inside, about 12 minutes.

In a small bowl, mix the olive oil, vinegar and mustard. Add pepper to taste.

Drizzle the oil mixture over the asparagus.

Makes 1 serving

Per serving: 89 calories, 5 g protein, 10 g carbohydrates, 5 g total fat, 5 g dietary fibre, 33 mg sodium

Roasted Tomatoes, Mushrooms and Red Onions

Keep track of the cooking time when making this recipe; otherwise the vegetables will shrivel and stick to the aluminium foil.

> 1 small plum tomato, chopped into 2.5 cm (1 in) pieces
>
> 40 g (1¼ oz) thickly sliced mushrooms
>
> ½ small red or sweet onion, thinly sliced
>
> 1 teaspoon olive oil
>
> 2 teaspoons sherry or red wine vinegar
>
> 1 teaspoon dried basil
>
> Ground black pepper

Preheat the oven to 200°C/400°F/gas 6.

In a large bowl, combine the tomato, mushrooms and onion. Add the oil, sherry or vinegar and basil. Mix well. Season with pepper to taste. Spread the vegetable mixture on a baking tray lined with aluminium foil and roast the vegetables until the onion slices are browned and all of the vegetables are tender, about 20 minutes.

Makes 1 serving

Per serving: 71 calories, 2 g protein, 6 g carbohydrates, 5 g total fat, 2 g dietary fibre, 36 mg sodium

Roasted Cauliflower and Red Peppers

Carrots, turnips or brussels sprouts can be substituted for the cauliflower in this recipe. If you use turnips or brussels sprouts, cook them for about 3 minutes in rapidly boiling water before roasting them – this cuts down on the roasting time.

> **100 g (3½ oz) cauliflower florets**
>
> **½ red pepper, sliced**
>
> **1 clove garlic, crushed**
>
> **1 teaspoon olive oil**
>
> **Olive oil cooking spray**
>
> **2 teaspoons dried basil or 2 tablespoons shredded fresh basil leaves**
>
> **¼ teaspoon ground black pepper**

Preheat the oven to 230°C/450°F/gas 8. Spread the cauliflower, pepper and garlic in a shallow baking tray lined with aluminium foil. Drizzle the vegetables with the olive oil, coat them with cooking spray and season them with the basil and black pepper. Roast until tender, about 12 minutes.

Makes 1 serving

Per serving: 84 calories, 3 g protein, 9 g carbohydrates, 5 g total fat, 4 g dietary fibre, 32 mg sodium

Smashed Peas

This recipe makes a nice starchy side dish for lamb, fish or ham. Peas are relatively high in starch compared to other vegetables. The result is a higher calorie content, so the portion sizes for this vegetable are slightly different.

> 230 g (8 oz) frozen peas, cooked according to package directions
>
> 1 teaspoon unsalted butter
>
> 4–5 fresh mint leaves, finely chopped
>
> 1 tablespoon low-sodium chicken or vegetable stock
>
> Salt (optional)
>
> Ground fresh black pepper

In a large bowl, using a potato masher or fork, smash the cooked peas with the butter, mint and stock until mushy. Add salt (if desired) and pepper to taste.

NOTE: If this is the only starch in the meal, you can increase the portion size to 200 g (7 oz) for women and 300 g (10½ oz) for men.

Per 100 g (3½ oz) serving (women): 111 calories, 5 g protein, 15 g carbohydrates, 3 g total fat, 6 g dietary fibre, 139 mg sodium

Per 200 g (7 oz) serving (men): 222 calories, 10 g protein, 31 g carbohydrates, 7 g total fat, 11 g dietary fibre, 278 mg sodium

OH HOT TOMATO!

Cherry tomatoes take on an intense sweetness when heated.

Olive oil cooking spray

1 teaspoon olive oil

1 tablespoon chopped shallots or the white ends of spring onions

150 g (5½ oz) cherry tomatoes

2 tablespoons chopped fresh parsley

Ground black pepper

In a frying pan liberally coated with cooking spray and set over medium heat, combine the oil and shallots or spring onions and cook for 2 minutes or until tender. Add the tomatoes and cook for 5 minutes or until slightly soft. Remove from heat and stir in the parsley. Season with pepper to taste.

Makes 1 serving

Per serving: 75 calories, 2 g protein, 7 g carbohydrates, 5 g total fat, 8 g dietary fibre, 36 mg sodium

Casablanca Onions

This dish is so tasty you will want to make extra.

> Cooking spray
>
> 1 teaspoon olive oil
>
> 2 sweet onions, thickly sliced
>
> ½ teaspoon ground coriander
>
> ¼ teaspoon cumin
>
> ¼ teaspoon cinnamon
>
> 115 g (4 oz) jarred tomato sauce or passata (optional: low-sodium variety)
>
> 60 ml (2 fl oz) low-sodium vegetable or chicken stock
>
> 1 tablespoon raisins or dried currants
>
> 1 bay leaf
>
> ½ teaspoon brown sugar
>
> Ground black pepper

Coat a frying pan with cooking spray and heat over low-medium heat. Add the olive oil and onions and sauté until soft, about 8 minutes. Remove the onions from the pan. Add the coriander, cumin and cinnamon to the frying pan and sauté for 1 minute.

Return the onions to the pan; add the tomato sauce, stock, raisins or currants and bay leaf; and cook for 30 minutes or until the sauce is thick and the onions are very tender.

Remove from heat and remove the bay leaf.

Stir in the sugar and season with pepper to taste.

Makes 1 serving

Per serving: 108 calories, 3 g protein, 20 g carbohydrates, 2 g total fat, 4 g dietary fibre, 18 mg sodium

SESAME MANGETOUT

We use the cooking method known as blanching *to preserve the bright green colour of the mangetout.*

> 1.7 litres (2¾ pt) water
>
> ½ tablespoon sea salt
>
> 60 g (2 oz) mangetout
>
> 1 teaspoon sesame oil
>
> 1 clove garlic, crushed
>
> 2.5 cm (1 in) piece fresh ginger, peeled and grated
>
> 1 teaspoon sesame seeds

In a very large pot, bring the water and salt to a rapid boil over high heat. Add the mangetout and boil for 1 minute. Remove from heat and pour the contents of the pot into a strainer. Rinse with very cold water to stop the cooking.

In a saucepan over medium heat, heat the sesame oil with the garlic and ginger and sauté until fragrant, about 2 minutes. Add the mangetout and sesame seeds and sauté for 1 minute, stirring frequently.

Makes 1 serving

Per serving: 93 calories, 3 g protein, 7 g carbohydrates, 6 g total fat, 2 g dietary fibre, 38 mg sodium

Cauliflower Soup

This soup is made from cauliflower florets and spring onions and is very simple to prepare.

> 240 ml (8 fl oz) low-sodium vegetable stock
>
> 1 tablespoon fresh lemon juice
>
> ½ medium fresh cauliflower, broken into florets, or 285 g (10 oz) frozen cauliflower
>
> ½ tablespoon olive oil
>
> 1 tablespoon chopped spring onion
>
> ¼ teaspoon ground black pepper
>
> Pinch of nutmeg

In a large pot over high heat, bring the stock and lemon juice to the boil. Reduce the heat to medium, add the cauliflower and cook until tender, about 10 minutes. Do not drain.

In a large nonstick frying pan, warm the oil over medium heat. Add the chopped spring onion. Cook until tender, about 5 minutes. Add the spring onion to the cauliflower and mix.

Purée the cauliflower until smooth, using a food processor or hand blender.

Stir in the pepper and nutmeg.

Makes 1 serving

Per serving: 87 calories, 6 g protein, 9 g carbohydrates, 4 g total fat, 4 g dietary fibre, 71 mg sodium

So Easy Tomato Sauce

The recipe makes 4 servings, so freeze the extra.

> 1 tablespoon olive oil
>
> 2–4 cloves garlic, crushed
>
> 1 large onion, chopped
>
> 100 g (3½ oz) chopped celery
>
> 75 g (2½ oz) sliced mushrooms (optional)
>
> 1 small carrot, grated
>
> 2 teaspoons Italian seasoning or 2 fresh basil leaves
>
> 1 tablespoon fresh thyme
>
> 2 x 400 g cans chopped whole tomatoes in juice
>
> Ground black pepper

Heat the oil in a large saucepan over low-medium heat.

Sauté the garlic, onion, celery and mushrooms (if desired) until soft, about 5 minutes.

Add the carrot, Italian seasoning or basil, and thyme. Cook until the carrot softens, about 5 minutes.

Add the tomatoes with their juice. Bring to the boil over high heat.

Reduce the heat to low-medium, cover and simmer until the sauce is thick, about 20 minutes. Season with pepper to taste.

Makes 4 servings

Per 240 ml (8 fl oz) serving: 101 calories, 3 g protein, 20 g carbohydrates, 4 g total fat, 4 g dietary fibre, 97 mg sodium

SALAD DRESSINGS

If you like to mix your own salad dressings, these delicious varieties can be used on raw salads as well as on cooked vegetables, pulses, meat and fish. One serving of each dressing is 1 tablespoon.

BALSAMIC VINAIGRETTE

1½ tablespoons olive oil

½ tablespoon balsamic vinegar

1 clove garlic, crushed

⅛ teaspoon salt

⅛ teaspoon black pepper

Combine all of the ingredients and mix well.

Per serving: 91 calories, 0 g protein, 0.5 g carbohydrates, 4 g total fat, 0 g dietary fibre, 117 mg sodium

FRENCH DRESSING

60 ml (2 fl oz) olive oil

1 tablespoon red wine vinegar

1 tablespoon lemon juice

1 teaspoon Dijon mustard

1 clove garlic, chopped

1 teaspoon dried tarragon

¼ teaspoon salt

¼ teaspoon white pepper

Combine all of the ingredients and mix well.

Per serving: 123 calories, 0 g protein, 0.8 g carbohydrates, 13 g total fat, 0 g dietary fibre, 162 mg sodium

ITALIAN DRESSING

60 ml (2 fl oz) olive oil

2 tablespoons balsamic vinegar

1 clove garlic, chopped

1 teaspoon dried basil

¼ teaspoon salt

¼ teaspoon ground black pepper

Combine all of the ingredients and mix well.

Per serving: 121 calories, 0 g protein, 0.5 g carbohydrates, 13 g total fat, 0 g dietary fibre, 146 mg sodium

JAPANESE DRESSING

1 tablespoon rice vinegar

2 tablespoons low-sodium soy sauce

½ teaspoon sesame oil

1 tablespoon chopped spring onion

½ tablespoon grated fresh ginger

½ teaspoon cayenne pepper

Combine all of the ingredients and mix well.

Per serving: 42 calories, 2 g protein, 2 g carbohydrates, 3 g total fat, 0 g dietary fibre, 1,067 mg sodium

MEXICAN DRESSING

2 tablespoons vegetable oil

2 tablespoons orange juice

1 chopped jalepeño chilli pepper or hot green chilli pepper (wear plastic gloves when handling)

1 tablespoon honey

1 teaspoon cumin

1 tablespoon chopped fresh coriander

Combine all of the ingredients and mix well.

Per serving: 82 calories, 1 g protein, 5 g carbohydrates, 7 g total fat, 0 g dietary fibre, 20 mg sodium

CHILLI AND LIME DRESSING

60 ml (2 fl oz) natural low-fat yogurt

Lambs lettuce

1 tablespoon chilli powder

1 tablespoon lime juice

¼ teaspoon salt (optional)

Combine all of the ingredients and mix well.

Per serving: 80 calories, 1 g protein, 3 g carbohydrates, 7 g total fat, 0.5 g dietary fibre, 57 mg sodium

Spanish Dressing

60 ml (2 fl oz) olive oil

1 tablespoon capers

2 tablespoons lemon juice

Grated rind from one lemon

1 clove garlic, chopped

1 tablespoon finely chopped green olives

Combine all of the ingredients and mix well.

Per serving: 91 calories, 0 g protein, 1 g carbohydrates, 10 g total fat, 0 g dietary fibre, 117 mg sodium

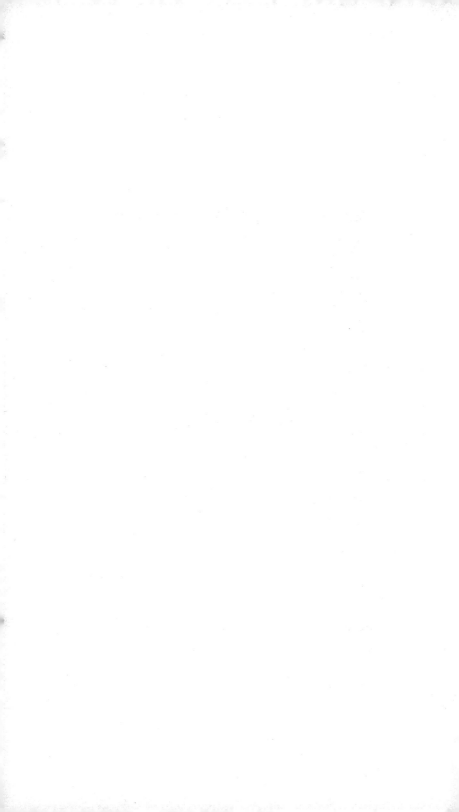

ENDNOTES

Chapter One: Solving the Carbohydrate Riddle

1. J. D. Fernstrom and D. V. Faller. 'Neutral Amino Acids in the Brain: Changes in Response to Food Ingestion', *Journal of Neurochemistry* 30 (1978): 1531–38.

2. J. D. Fernstrom and R. J. Wurtman. 'Brain Serotonin Content: Physiological Dependence on Plasma Tryptophan Levels', *Science* 173 (1971): 149–52.

3.——. 'Brain Serotonin Content: Increase Following Ingestion of Carbohydrate Diet', *Science* 174 (1971): 1023–25.

4.——. 'Brain Serotonin Content: Physiological Regulation by Plasma Neutral Amino Acids', *Science* 178 (1972): 414–16.

5. A. Amer et al. '5-Hydroxytryptophan Raises Plasma 5-HTP Levels in Humans and Rats and Suppresses Food Intake by Hypophagic and Stressed Rats', *Pharmacology, Biochemistry and Behavior* 77 (2004): 137–43.

6. J. J. Wurtman, P. L. Moses, and R. J. Wurtman. 'Prior Carbohydrate Consumption Affects the Amount of Carbohydrate that Rats Choose to Eat', *Journal of Nutrition* 113 (1983): 70–78.

7. J. J. Wurtman and R. J. Wurtman. 'Drugs that Enhance Central Serotoninergic Transmission Diminish Elective Carbohydrate Consumption by Rats', *Life Sciences 24 (1979): 895–904.*

8. S. Nishizawa et al. 'Differences Between Males and Females in Rates of Serotonin Synthesis in Human Brain', Proceedings of the National Academy of Sciences USA 94 (1997): 5308–13.

9. R. Deshmukh and K. Franco. 'Managing Weight Gain as a Side Effect of Antidepressant Therapy', *Cleveland Clinic Journal of Medicine* 70 (2003): 614–23.

10. J. M. Ferguson. 'SSRI Antidepressant Medications: Adverse Effects and Tolerability', *Primary Care Companion Journal of Clinical Psychiatry* 3 (2001): 22–27.

11. T. L. Schwartz et al. 'Psychiatric Medication-Induced Obesity: Treatment Options,' *Obesity Review* 5 (2004): 233–38.

12. J. J. Wurtman et al. 'The Effect of a Novel Dietary Intervention on Weight Loss in Psychotropic Drug-Induced Obesity', *Psychopharmacology Bulletin* 36, no. 3 (Summer 2002): 55–59.

Chapter Five: Snack Your Way to Serotonin Power

1. R. J. Wurtman and J. J. Wurtman. 'Carbohydrates and Depression,' *Scientific American* 260, no. 1 (January 1989): 68–75.

2. J. J. Wurtman et al. 'Carbohydrate Craving in Obese People: Suppression by Treatments Affecting Serotoninergic Transmission,' *International Journal of Eating Disorders* 1 (1981): 2–15.

Chapter Seven: Change Your Body

1. M. L. Klem et al. 'A Descriptive Study of Individuals Successful at Long-Term Maintenance of Substantial Weight Loss,' *American Journal of Clinical Nutrition* 66 (1997): 239–46.

2. J. A. Levine et al. 'Interindividual Variation in Posture Allocation: Possible Role in Human Obesity,' *Science* 307 (2005): 584–86.

3. K. Helliker. 'Yet Another Reason to Go to the Gym: How Exercise Can Help Fight Depression,' *The Wall Street Journal*, May 10, 2005: D1.

INDEX

Underscored references indicate boxed text.

A

Acid reflux, 161–62
Activity, daily. *See also* Exercise
  ideas for keeping busy, 147
  pedometer to monitor, 96, 137
  phone headset for mobility, 106
  weight loss and, 95
Aerobic exercise
  benefits of, 97
  increasing intensity of, 139, 145
  strength training with, 96
  types of, 98
  weekly prescription, 97, 98–99
Afternoons
  fatigue and, 70
  home stress during, 43
  mood and, 69–71
  overeating during, 137
  serotonin levels during, 69–71
Airport food options, 119
Alcoholic drinks, 91, 158
Anniversaries, eating and, 145
Antidepressants
  appetite and, 19, 23, 33
  carbohydrate cravings and, 3,
    28–30
  changes to, and stalled weight,
    168
  diet effectiveness and, 48
  side effects of, 20
  weight gain and, 4, 19–21
  weight loss despite using, 31–32
Appetite
  antidepressants and, 19, 23
  and the brain, 7–9
  exercise and, 110
  lack of sleep and, 44

SAD and, 92
  self-test for assessing, 25–26
  serotonin and, 4, 7, 11–13, 33
  uncontrolled, and weight gain, 26
  vs. hunger, 25–26
Appetizers, at receptions, 148
Appliances, kitchen, 180
Asian-inspired recipes
  Asian Chicken Wrap, 200
  Asian Rice and Prawn Salad, 221
  Curried Thai Sweet Potato and
    Chicken Soup, 229
  Japanese Dressing, 255
  Nam Chinese Noodles with Tofu
    or Chicken, 232–33
  Pad Thai Salad, 210
  Seared Spicy Tuna Salad, 202–3
  Sushi Rice Salad, 212
Asian restaurants
  Chinese, 115
  Indian, 117
  Japanese, 116
  Thai, 117
Asparagus
  Roasted Asparagus Spears with
    Vinaigrette, 245
Asthma, exercise and, 99, 110
Awards dinners, food at, 124–25

B

Barley
  Barley and Corn Salad with
    Chicken, 241
Beano, 94
Beans
  digestion and, 94

recipes
  Corn Burritos, 231
  Meat, Rice and Beans with a
    Kick, 235
  Red Lentil and Cauliflower
    Curry, 219
  Turkey Lentil Stew with
    Greens, 240
Beef
  Beef Stir-Fry, 205
  Cheeseburger, 194
  Meat, Rice and Beans with a Kick,
    235
  Mushroom Burger, 213–14
  Pasta with Meat and Mushroom-
    Tomato Ragu, 228
  Polenta with Mushrooms and
    Meat, 226
  Roast Beef Roll-Up, 239
  Sirloin Steak with Mushrooms,
    195
  Very Fast Beef and Broccoli with
    Rice, 242
Beverages
  alcoholic, 91, 158
  coffee and coffee drinks, 75, 163
  high-calorie, 157
  juice alternatives, 163
  tea, 75
Bingeing
  carbohydrate deprivation and, 11, 14
  Premenstrual Syndrome and, 160
  to relieve stress, 16–17
  on snacks, 160
Birthday parties
  eating moderately at, 159
  restaurant choices at, 123–24
  temptations at, 37
Blanching, as cooking method, 189
Boredom
  at dinner meetings, 159
  eating and, 151
Brain
  appetite regulation and, 7–9
  carbohydrate cravings and, 26, 70
  serotonin connection with, 5–7, 70
  tryptophan and, 6
Bread
  fresh, as good snack, <u>67</u>
  portion sizes, by phase, 91

Breakfast
  grab-and-go, <u>182</u>
  phase 1
    guidelines for, 75–76
    sample menus, 79–81
  phase 2
    guidelines for, 75–76, 82
    sample menus, 84–85
  phase 3
    guidelines for, 75–76, 87
    protein at, 153
    sample menus, 88–89
  protein and, 90
  quick trick ideas for, 181–85
  on sleep-in Sundays, 93
Breathing
  as calming mini-break, 143
  during stretching, 103
Broccoli
  Fast Creamy Broccoli Rice, 214
  Very Fast Beef and Broccoli with
    Rice, 242
Buckwheat
  Buckwheat and Farfalle Pasta, 220
Buffets, prepaid, 158
Bulgur
  Tabouli, 218
Burgers
  Cheeseburger, 194
  Mushroom Burger, 212–13

C

Cabbage
  Coleslaw, 244
Cajun recipes
  Cajun Prawn Stew, 227
Calories
  exercise and, 95
  saved, by eating lean, <u>128</u>
Carbohydrates
  afternoon cravings for, 70–72
  antidepressants and, 19–21, 33
  bingeing and, 160
  complex, 5
  cooking methods, 186–189
  deprivation, effects of, 7–9, 11, 14
  eaten with protein, 15
  love-hate relationship with, 3

phase 1 guidelines, for
  breakfast, 75
  dinner, 77–78
phase 2 guidelines, for
  breakfast, 75
  dinner, 83
phase 3 guidelines, for
  breakfast, 87
  dinner, 87
popular beliefs about, 4, 34
serotonin and
  emotions and, 29–30
  high-fat carbohydrates, 17–18
simple, 4–5
as stress reliever, 17, <u>43</u>
types of, 4–5
Cardiovascular health
  exercise and, 97, 100
Caribbean recipes
  Spicy Caribbean Potato Chunks
    with Steak or Pork, 230
Carrots
  Carrot and Cumin Soup, 243
Cauliflower
  Cauliflower Soup, 252
  Red Lentil and Cauliflower Curry,
    219
  Roasted Cauliflower and Red
    Peppers, 247
Change
  forming new habits, 55–56
  realistic, 51–53, <u>55</u>
  setting priorities and, <u>56</u>
Chicken
  Asian Chicken Wrap, 200
  Asian Rice Salad, 221
  Barley and Corn Salad with
    Chicken, 241
  Chicken Soup in a Hurry, 225
  Couscous with Courgette and
    Chicken, 237
  Crusty Bread Salad with Chicken,
    222–23
  Curried Thai Sweet Potato and
    Chicken Soup, 229
  Lemony Chicken, 198
  Nam Chinese Noodles with Tofu
    or Chicken, 232–33
  Polenta with Mushrooms and
    Meat, 226

  Roast Chicken and Vegetables, 208
  Stir-Fry, 205
  Sweet and Spicy Chicken, 204
Chinese restaurants, 115
Chocolate, 129
Clothes
  discarding, if too big, 147, <u>169</u>
  with elastic waistbands, 50
  for exercise, 50, 150
  snug, to avoid overeating, 151
Coffee
  drinks, calories and, 163
  in place of dessert, 113
Coffee shop temptations, 37
Commitment to weight loss, 47,
    148–49
Condiments, 91
Courgette
  Couscous with Courgette and
    Chicken, 237
  Crusty Bread Salad with Chicken,
    222–23
Couscous
  recipes
    Couscous with Lamb, 234
    Couscous with Courgette and
      Chicken, 237
Cravings, carbohydrate
  antidepressants and, 19–21
  daily carbohydrates for, 13
  due to stress, 16–17
  eating dinner early, 148
  in the evening, 82
  SAD and, 92
  serotonin and, 7–9, 26
  snacks to reduce, 10–11
Cross-training, 98

D

Dairy products
  milk, 90
  yogurt, 75
Depression, clinical
  exercise and, 96
  in the UK, 19–20
Desserts
  coffee in place of, 113
  at restaurants, 113

Diabetes
  doctor's guidance for, 21
  exercise and, 96
Diaries, food. *See* Journals, food
Dieting
  determining reasons for, 49
  reluctance to mention, 48
  when to start, 57
Diets. *See also* Good Mood Diet
  high-protein, for weight-loss, 28
  high-protein, high-fat, 13–14
  high-protein, low-carb, 26
  mindset for success, 36, 36, 45
Dining out. *See also* Restaurants
  with business clients, 58
  on holiday, 57
Dinner
  advice about
    dietary fat, 90
    protein, 93, 152
  carbohydrate suggestions for, 78
  early, to satisfy cravings, 148
  ideas for
    lasagne, 94
    pizza, 185
    quick tricks, 185
  phase 1
    guidelines, 74–76
    recipes, 210–20
    sample menus, 79–81
  phase 2
    guidelines, 82–83
    recipes, 221–42
    sample menus, 84–86
    soups, 94
  phase 3
    guidelines, 86–87
    recipes, 221–42
    sample menus, 88–89
Disability and exercise, 110
Dressings, salad
  Balsamic Vinaigrette, 254
  Chilli and Lime Dressing, 256
  French Dressing, 254
  Italian Dressing, 255
  Japanese Dressing, 255
  Mexican Dressing, 256
  Spanish Dressing, 257
  Vinaigrette, 221, 238
Drinks. *See* Beverages

E

Eating. *See also* Overeating
  appetite vs. hunger, 25
  automatic, 161
  coping with special situations
    air travel, 119
    awards dinner, 124
    birthday dinners, 123
    end-of-the-week drinks,
      123
    evening workouts, 120
    family gatherings, 127, 159
    job meetings, 121
    wedding receptions,
      120
  emotional, 17, 29–30
  inattentive, 158
  late at night, 162–63
  as main pleasure, 44
  measuring food, 143, 150, 158
  mood and, 33
  in restaurants, 112–18
  stress and, 16–18, 28–29, 126
  tasting for enjoyment, 145
Eggs
  Tuna, Turkey and Egg Salad, 196
  whites of, for protein, 183
Emotions
  food as comfort, 17
  overeating and, 29–30
  self-test for assessing, 29
Excuses, 47, 103–5, 108, 148
Exercise
  aerobic. *See* Aerobic Exercise
  antidepressants and, 31
  appetite and, 110–11
  backup exercise plan, 141
  benefits of, 95–97
  boredom and, 144
  cardiovascular health and, 96, 100
  cross-training, 97–98
  equipment for
    clothes, 49
    heart-rate monitors, 99, 148
    pedometers, 96, 137
    shoes for, 100
    treadmills, 104
    TV programmes and videos,
      105, 106

excuses not to, 103–5, <u>108</u>, 148
fears about, 146
with friends, 104
intensity, 99, <u>101</u>
during maintenance, 111
motivation for, 105–6
multitasking during, 141
planning for, 142
programme requirements, 99–100
with resistance. *See* Strength
    Training
special circumstances
  asthma, 110
  disability, 110
  illness, 152
  knee trouble, 59
  weather, 108–9
  when fatigued, <u>103</u>
special situations
  family obligations, 126–27
stalled weight and, 156
stretching and, 102–3
success stories, 106–7
variety and, 151
Expectations, realistic, 51–53

F

Family
  Sunday dinners, 127
  unsupportive, 126, 146
  weight loss together, 55
Fast-food chains, eating at, 118
Fat, body
  calculating fat-burning zone, 99
  strength training and, 97–98
Fat, dietary
  healthiest choices, 90
  in restaurant foods, 112, 113, 117
Fatigue
  exercising despite, <u>103</u>
  in late afternoon, 70
Fennel
  Prawn and Fennel Stir-Fry, 201
Fish
  Crusty Trusty Trout, 206
  Fish and Roasted Acorn Squash
    Stuffed with Wild Rice Mix,
    236

Fish with Barbecue Sauce, 207
  Halibut with Peppers, 199
  Niçoise-Inspired Tuna and Herbed
    Potato Salad, 238–39
  Pasta Shells with Smoked Salmon,
    224
  Sautéed Scallops, 193
  Seared Spicy Tuna Salad,
    202–3
  Tuna Chopped Salad, 209
  Warm Salmon Salad, 197
Fizzy drinks
  as ineffective snack, 73
  stalled weight and, 157
Flexibility, stretching for, 102
Flour, refined, 93
Food courts at shopping centres, 39
Food labels, 65, 67, 138
Foods. *See also specific foods*
  for breakfast
    in all phases, <u>75</u>
    quick trick ideas, 181–82
  calorie comparison of, <u>128</u>
  for dinner
    quick trick ideas, 185
  for lunch
    in phase 1, 77
    quick trick ideas, 181–85
  at restaurants, 112–19
  sampling non-diet, 146
  snack
    for phase 3, 67
    for phases 1 and 2, 66
  spicy, 91
  to stock, for
    quick meals, 177–79
    quick snacks, 179
  sweet
    serotonin and, 70
  tasting for enjoyment, 145
Freezer foods to stock, 177
Friends
  exercising with, 104
  as support, 54, 58
  unsupportive, 146
Fructose
  glucose conversion from, 5
  serotonin and, 73
Fruits
  as dessert, at restaurants, 113

glucose conversion from, 5
one a day, 76

G

Gas, intestinal, and beans, 94
Gels, energy, 70, 73
Gender, serotonin and, <u>15</u>
Glucose, carbohydrates and, 4–5
Glycaemic index, 73
Glycogen, 5
Goals for weight-loss
  patience and, 144–45
  setting realistic goals, 51–52
Good Mood Diet
  dietary fats in, 90
  excuses and, 148
  getting started, 49, 133–34
  how it works, 11–13
  phase 1
    breakfast guidelines, 75–76
    dinner guidelines, 77
    lunch guidelines, 77–78
    meals and snacks outline, 74
    sample menus, 79–81
    summary, <u>74</u>, 79
    week-by-week guide to, 133–36
  phase 2
    breakfast guidelines, 75–76, 82
    dinner guidelines, 82–83
    lunch guidelines, 83
    sample menus, 84–86
    summary, <u>82</u>, 84
    week-by-week guide to, 136–44
  phase 3
    alcoholic drinks in, 91
    celebrating your success, 154
    guidelines for, 86–87
    sample menus, 88–89
    snacks, 153
    summary, <u>86</u>, 87
    week-by-week guide to, 144–53
  snacks, 63–74
  special populations
    diabetics, <u>21</u>
    nursing mothers, 91
    teenagers, 93
  stalled, reasons for, 157–63
  troubleshooting, 155–63
  week-by-week guide to, 133–54

Grains, whole
  experimenting with, <u>220</u>
  for nutritional value, 93
  vs. sugary foods, 72–73
Greens
  Turkey Lentil Stew with Greens,
    240
Grilling
  as cooking method, 190

H

Habits, forming new, 55–56
Health clubs, 139
Heart. *See* Cardiovascular health
Heart-rate monitors, 99, 148
Hobbies for busy hands, 137
Holidays, eating and, 145
Home
  afternoon overeating, 43, 140
  portion sizes at, 138
  temptations at, 38
Hunger
  false signals of, 161
  real, 24–25
  vs. appetite, 25–26

I

Illness, exercise and, 152
Indian-inspired recipes
  Indian Roasted Potato Chunks
    with Mint, 216–17
  Red Lentil and Cauliflower Curry,
    219
Indian restaurants, 117
Injury prevention
  strength training and, 101–2
  stretching and, 102
Insulin
  blood sugar regulation and, 73
  carbohydrates and, 4, 6
  fructose and, 73
Italian-inspired recipes
  Crusty Bread Salad with Chicken,
    222–23
  Italian Dressing, 255
  Italian Flag Salad, 211
Italian restaurants, 114–15

J

Japanese restaurants, 116
Journals, food
    during maintenance, 167, 172
    to pinpoint trouble spots, <u>155</u>
    as weight loss technique, 54
Juice
    alternatives to, 163
    stalled weight loss and, 157

K

Kitchen equipment
    appliances, <u>180</u>
    food scales, 134
    measuring scales, 144
Knees, bad, and exercise, 59

L

Lactose, 4
Lamb
    Couscous with Lamb, 234
Lasagne, 94
Leftovers temptations, 138
Lentils
    Red Lentil and Cauliflower Curry,
        219
    Turkey Lentil Stew with Greens,
        240
Lifestyle change, <u>56</u>
Lunch
    bringing from home, 183
    grab-and-go, <u>184</u>
    as hot meal, 184
    phase 1
        guidelines, 77
        recipes, 193–99
        sample menus, 79–81
    phase 2
        guidelines, 83
        recipes, 200–9
        sample menus, 84–85
    phase 3
        guidelines, 87
        recipes, 200–9
        sample menus, 88–89

    quick trick ideas for, 182–84
    stressful afternoon meetings and,
        127–28

M

Maintenance of weight goal
    balancing food and exercise,
        166–68
    checklist, 173
    exercise and, 169–70
    guidelines, by week, 167–68
    portion sizes, 172
    rewarding yourself, 172
    rules for, 171–72
    snacks, 165–66
    staying vigilant, 172
    stress and, 166
    weigh-ins, 167, 172
    weight gain and, <u>168</u>
Meals. *See also* Breakfast; Dinner;
        Lunch
    foods to stock for, 177–78
    planning, as new habit, 142
    quick trick ideas for, 181–86
    seasonal adjustments to, 145
    skipping, 158
Mental attitude
    excuses
        not to exercise, 103–5, <u>108</u>, 148
        not to lose weight, <u>47</u>
    ideas for the weight-loss journey,
        145
    overcoming temptations, 40–41
    prioritizing commitments, 148
    for weight loss, 35, <u>36</u>, 45
Menus, sample, for
    phase 1, 79–81
    phase 2, 84–85
    phase 3, 88–89
Mexican-inspired recipes
    Chilli and Lime Dressing, 256
    Corn Burritos, 231
    Mexican Dressing,
        256
Mexican restaurants, 116
Microwaving
    potatoes, 187
    protein food sources, 186
    vegetables, 190

Middle Eastern recipes
  Tabouli, 217
Milk, 90
Millet, 220
Mirrors, full-length, 154
Monosodium glutamate (MSG),
  116
Mood
  antidepressants and, 32
  eating to improve, 33
  exercise and, 96
  in late afternoon, 70
  SAD and, 160
  serotonin and, 16–17, 18
Motivation
  to exercise, 103
  for weight loss, 49–50
MSG, in Japanese food, 116
Mushrooms
  Mushroom Burger, 212–13
  Pasta with Meat and Mushroom-
    Tomato Ragu, 228
  Polenta with Mushrooms and
    Meat, 226
  Roasted Tomatoes, Mushrooms
    and Red Onions, 246
Mustards, for flavour, 186

N

Nursing mothers, 91, 111
Nutritional value
  of coloured vegetables, 140
  food labels and, 65, 67, 138–39
  of snacks, by phase, 63–64
  of whole grains, 191

O

Obesity, inactivity and, 96
Onions
  Casablanca Onions, 250
  Roasted Tomatoes, Mushrooms
    and Red Onions, 246
  Spaghetti with Roasted Courgette
    and Onion, 215
Osteoporosis, exercise and, 96
Overeating
  boredom and, 151

cleaning your plate and, 159
  emotions and, 29–30
  feeling deprived and, 161
  lack of sleep and, 44
  late afternoons at home, 140
  long winter evenings and, 140
  multitasking and, 158
  portion sizes and, 158
  reasons for, 19–20, 160–61
  recognizing causes of, 147
  routine changes and, 161
  snacks, 159–60
  snug clothes and, 151
  time and, 160–61

P

Pancakes
  Potato Pancakes, 218
Pantry foods to stock, 178, 180
Pasta
  lasagne, modified, 94
  leftovers, reheating, 188
  recipes
    Buckwheat and Farfalle Pasta,
      220
    Nam Chinese Noodles with
      Tofu or Chicken, 232–33
    Pasta Shells with Smoked
      Salmon, 224
    Pasta with Meat and
      Mushroom-Tomato Ragu,
      228
    Spaghetti with Roasted
      Courgette and Onion, 215
  toppings for, 188
  whole grain, 93
Peas
  Sesame Mangetout, 251
  Smashed Peas, 248
Pedometers, 96, 137
Peppers
  Crusty Bread Salad with Chicken,
    222–23
  Halibut with Peppers, 199
  Meat, Rice and Bean with a Kick,
    235
  Roasted Cauliflower and Red
    Peppers, 247

Phones
    alarms, setting for snacks, 54
    headsets for mobility, <u>106</u>
Pilates, 101
Pizza, as dinner choice, 185
Planning
    for exercise, 144
    meals, as new habit, 141
    for weight loss, 51–53
PMS
    bingeing and, 160
    serotonin and, 10, 29
Polenta
    baking, <u>189</u>
    cooking, 189
    Polenta with Mushrooms and
        Meat, 226
Pork
    Spicy Caribbean Potato Chunks
        with Steak or Pork, 230
Portion sizes
    at home, 148, 159
    during maintenance, 172
    measuring food, 143, 150,
        158
    in recipes, 192
    at restaurants, 112, 138, 158
    snacks, measuring, 159
    stalled weight and, 157–59
Posture, strength training and, 101
Potatoes
    baking methods, 186–88
    recipes
        Indian Roasted Potato Chunks
            with Mint, 216–17
        Niçoise-Inspired Tuna and
            Herbed Potato Salad, 238–39
        Potato Pancakes, 216
        Spicy Caribbean Potato Chunks
            with Steak or Pork, 230
        twice-baked, 188
    toppings for, <u>187</u>
Potatoes, sweet
    Curried Thai Sweet Potato and
        Chicken Soup, 229
Prawns
    Asian Rice and Prawn Salad, 221
    Cajun Prawn Stew, 227
    Prawn and Fennel Stir-Fry, 201
    Stir-Fry, 205

Pre-meal carbohydrate intake, 11–13
Premenstrual Syndrome (PMS)
    bingeing and, 160
    serotonin and, 10, 29
Protein bars, 122, 136, <u>184</u>
Protein, dietary
    at breakfast, 90, 152
    with carbohydrates, 15
    cooking methods, 186
    at dinner, 93, 153
    high, in popular diets, 13–14, 25
    nursing mothers and, 91
    phase 1
        foods for breakfast, 75
        foods for lunch, 77
    phase 2 and 3
        foods for breakfast, 82
        foods for lunch, 83
    serotonin and, 5–6, 15
    in soups, <u>225</u>
Prozac, 19

Q

Quinoa, <u>220</u>

R

Refrigerator foods to stock, 179
Resistance training. *See* Strength
    training
Restaurants
    calorie comparison of foods at,
        <u>128</u>
    choices, by cuisine type
        Chinese, 115
        fast-food chains, 118–19
        Indian, 117
        Italian, 114–15
        Japanese, 116
        Mexican, 116
        steak houses, 117–18
        Thai, 117
    custom ordering at, 113
    fat content of, 114, 139
    portion sizes at, 113, 138, 158
Rewarding yourself
    exercise and, 106–7
    by having fun, 150

in healthy ways, 38–39, 40
in non-food ways, 142, 170, 172
weekly, 50
Rice
  brown, 93, 191
  recipes
    Asian Rice and Prawn Salad,
      221
    Corn Burritos, 231
    Fast Creamy Broccoli Rice, 214
    Fish and Roasted Acorn Squash
      Stuffed with Wild Rice Mix,
      236
    Meat, Rice and Bean with a
      Kick, 235
    Sushi Rice Salad, 213
    Very Fast Beef and Broccoli
      with Rice, 242

S

SAD, 160
Salads
  dressing recipes, 254–57
  phase 1 dinners
    Pad Thai Salad, 210
    Sushi Rice Salad, 213
    Tabouli, 217
  phase 1 lunches
    Tuna, Turkey and Egg Salad,
      196
    Warm Salmon Salad, 197
  phase 2 and 3 dinners
    Asian Rice and Prawn Salad,
      221
    Barley and Corn Salad with
      Chicken, 241
    Crusty Bread Salad with
      Chicken, 222–23
    Niçoise-Inspired Tuna and
      Herbed Potato Salad, 238–39
  phase 2 and 3 lunches
    Seared Spicy Tuna Salad,
      202–3
    Tuna Chopped Salad, 209
  salad bars, for lunch, 153, 190
  as vegetable side dishes
    Coleslaw, 244
    Italian Flag Salad, 211
    Lemon Garlic Spinach, 244

Roasted Tomatoes, Mushrooms
    and Red Onions, 246
Salmon
  Pasta Shells with Smoked Salmon,
    224
  Warm Salmon Salad, 197
Salt substitutes, 192
Sauces
  for flavour, 92–93
  recipes
    Barbecue Sauce, 207
    So Easy Tomato Sauce, 253
    Yogurt Dipping Sauce, 217
Sautéing vegetables, 190
Scales
  bathroom, 50
Scallops
  Sautéed Scallops, 193
Seafood
  Cajun Prawn Stew, 227
  Crusty Trusty Trout, 206
  Fish and Roasted Acorn Squash
    Stuffed with Wild Rice Mix,
    236
  Fish with Barbecue Sauce, 207
  Halibut with Peppers, 199
  Niçoise-Inspired Tuna and Herbed
    Potato Salad, 238–39
  Prawn and Fennel Stir-Fry, 201
  Sautéed Scallops, 193
  Seared Spicy Tuna Salad, 202–3
  Tuna Chopped Salad, 209
  Warm Salmon Salad, 197
Seasonal affective disorder (SAD),
  160
Seasons. *See also* SAD
  adjusting menus for, 145
  exercise, in winter, 108–9
  long winter evenings, 140
  weight gain and, 168
Selective serotonin reuptake
    inhibitors (SSRIs), 19
  finding meaningful activities,
    142
  making time for yourself, 42, 153
  self-commitment, 56
Serotonin
  appetite and
    research results, 7–9
    serotonin as switch, 4, 7, 11–13,
      33

behavioural changes and, 71
as brain chemical, 4
carbohydrates and
   cravings, 9, 26
   physiology of, 4
in late afternoon, 71–72
mood and, <u>15</u>, 16–17, 33, 70
Premenstrual Syndrome and, 10,
   29
as stress reliever, <u>18</u>, 18, <u>43</u>
tryptophan and, 5–6
women and, <u>15</u>
Serotrim drink
  history of, 10
  in place of snack food, 10
Shakes, protein, <u>184</u>
Sherry, in soups, <u>225</u>
Shift work, overeating and, 161
Shoes, for exercise, 100
Sleep
  advice for a good night's, <u>162</u>
  exercise and, 96, <u>103</u>
  overeating and, 44, 160
Snacks
  afternoon need for, 70–72
  chocolate, 129
  daily schedules for, 63–64
  foods to stock for, 180
  how to snack, 64–65
  measuring, 158
  missed, 68
  nutritional value of, 65
  overeating of, 159–60
  phase 1
    sample menus, 79–81
    suggestions for, 66
  phase 2
    sample menus, 84–86
    suggestions for, 66
  phase 3
    sample menus, 88–89
    suggestions for, 67
  portion sizes, 148
  post-snack activities, 69
  Serotrim drink, 10–11
  setting phone alarm for, 54
  sweet, 67, 72–73
  travel and, <u>71</u>, 119
  as treatment, not treat, 63
  as willpower booster, <u>71</u>
Social functions

asking friends for help, 58
take dishes to share, 140
temptations at, 36
Sodium, in diet, 193
Soups
  low-fat, as meal basis, <u>225</u>
  in diet phases, 94
  recipes
    Carrot and Cumin Soup, 243
    Cauliflower Soup, 252
    Chicken Soup in a Hurry, 225
    Curried Thai Sweet Potato and
      Chicken Soup, 229
    Turkey Lentil Stew with
      Greens, 240
Spaghetti
  Spaghetti with Roasted Courgette
    and Onion, 215
Spicy foods, 91
Spinach
  Italian Flag Salad, 211
Squash
  Fish and Roasted Acorn Squash
    Stuffed with Wild Rice Mix,
    236
Starches, 5
Steak
  Sirloin Steak with Mushrooms,
    195
  Spicy Caribbean Potato Chunks
    with Steak or Pork, 230
Steak houses, 117–18
Steaming vegetables, 190
Stews
  Turkey Lentil Stew with Greens,
    240
Stir-frys
  as cooking method, 186
  recipes
    Beef Stir-Fry, 205
    Prawn and Fennel Stir-Fry, 201
Strength training
  aerobic exercise with, 96
  benefits of, 101
  body fat and, 96
  defined, 101
  flabby body and, 111
  intensity of, 146, 149
  types of, 101
  weekly prescription, 101–2, 103
  weights for, 97

Stress
eating and, 16–18, 29–30, 127
relief of, with food, 18
serotonin and, 32, _42_
situational
afternoon business meetings,
127–28
dieting concerns, 45
family-related, 92, 166, 172–73
food as sole pleasure, 44
lack of sleep, 44
late afternoon at home, 44
no time for myself, 44
'no time to shop' stress, 44
overworking, 42–43
Sundays with nothing to do, 44
suggestions for reducing, 45
yoga and, _105_
Stretching
benefits of, 102
types of, 102
weekly prescription, 102–3
Sucrose, 4
Sugars
as simple carbohydrates, 4
vs. sugar substitutes, _13_
Sundays
with nothing to do, 44
sleeping late on, 93
Supermarkets
foods to stock, 178–80
'no time to shop' stress, 44
temptations at, 37–38, 40
Support
asking for, 48, 58, 136
coping with little, 48, 126
husband–wife weight loss, 55
mutual, by e-mail, 54
unsupportive family, 126, 146
Sweetcorn
as dinner carbohydrate, 78, 83
recipes
Barley and Corn Salad with
Chicken, 241
Corn Burritos, 231

T

Teenagers, Good Mood Diet and,
92–93

Temptations
20-second rule for, 40
leftovers, 138
seven mental strategies for, 40–41
at social functions, 39
in a typical week, 37–40
Tests, self, about
antidepressants, 31
appetite vs. hunger, 25–26
emotions, 29
high-protein diets, 28
Thai restaurants, 117
Time
overeating and, 161
to spend alone, finding, 153
Tofu
Asian Rice Salad, 221
Nam Chinese Noodles with Tofu
or Chicken, 232–33
Stir-Fry, 205
Tomatoes
Oh Hot Tomato!, 249
Roasted Tomatoes, Mushrooms
and Red Onions, 246
So Easy Tomato Sauce, 253
Toppings, for
baked potatoes, _187_
pasta, 188
Travel
airport food options, 119
snacks and, _71_, 122
Treadmills, 104
Treats, 151–52
Trout
Crusty Trusty Trout, 206
Tryptophan
carbohydrates and, 4
foods containing, 5
process for entering the brain, 6
serotonin production and, 5
Tuna
Niçoise-Inspired Tuna and Herbed
Potato Salad, 238–39
Seared Spicy Tuna Salad, 202–3
Tuna Chopped Salad, 209
Tuna, Turkey and Egg Salad, 196
Turkey
Polenta with Mushrooms and
Meat, 226
Meat, Rice and Beans with a Kick,
235